Praise for *Mindfulness for Life*

"This book is a trustworthy and user-friendly roadmap for navigating the ups and downs of life with increasing degrees of intentionality, wisdom, and, above all, agency. By listening deeply to and implementing even some of the vast repertoire of offerings here, you can come home to and befriend the unique beauty of who you are and the life that is yours to live."   —Jon Kabat-Zinn, PhD, founder of
Mindfulness-Based Stress Reduction; author of
Wherever You Go, There You Are—30th Anniversary Edition

"This book is not just about inner change; it is about how we live our lives. Dr. Kuyken provides tools for making a critical shift from judgment, blame, and aversion to curiosity and kindness. His skillful guidance allows us to make—and commit to—small shifts that can help us become the flourishing, engaged, and responsive people we long to be."
—Christina Feldman, author of *Boundless Heart*

"Internationally renowned psychologist Willem Kuyken explains why and how mindfulness practice can help you 'light up your life with a sense of reconnection and love.' Whether you are new to mindfulness or have been practicing for years, this is a book to treasure—step by step, it reveals ways to reorient toward your deepest values and lead a life worth living."   —Mark Williams, DPhil, coauthor of
The Mindful Way Through Depression

"This thoughtful and kind scientist offers a wise framework for a life well lived. The book creates opportunities to cultivate a better friendship with your body and mind."   —Eric B. Loucks, PhD, author of
The Mindful College Student

MINDFULNESS FOR LIFE

Also from Willem Kuyken

Mindfulness
for Life

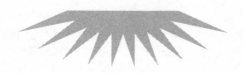

Willem Kuyken, PhD

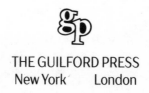

THE GUILFORD PRESS
New York   London

Library of Congress Cataloging-in-Publication Data

Names: Kuyken, W. (Willem), 1968– author.
Title: Mindfulness for life / Willem Kuyken.
Description: New York : The Guilford Press, [2024] | Includes index.
Identifiers: LCCN 2024022185 | ISBN 9781462543977 (paperback)
    | ISBN 9781462555260 (hardcover)
Subjects: LCSH: Mindfulness (Psychology) | Meditation--Therapeutic use. |
    BISAC: PSYCHOLOGY / Mental Health | SOCIAL SCIENCE / Social Work
Classification: LCC BF637.M56 K89 2024 | DDC 158.1/3—dc23/eng/20240703
LC record available at *https://lccn.loc.gov/2024022185*

To Zoe and Ava Cohen Kuyken

Contents

Audio downloads for many of the practices are available
at *mindfulnessforlife.uk* and *www.guilford.com/kuyken2-materials*.

Acknowledgments

There are a pair of 14th-century stone effigies in Chichester Cathedral lying side by side, a male knight, in full armor, and a woman, wearing a gown, veil, and mantle—most strikingly, they've removed their gloves to hold hands. Inspired by these two figures, Philip Larkin wrote a poem, "An Arundel Tomb," that ends with the line "What will survive of us is love." Friends and family have held my hand and supported me on a lifelong journey of befriending myself so I could better embody the thesis of this book. Thank you for your love.

Thanks to Halley Cohen, without whom I would never have been able to contemplate, let alone write, this book; Ava and Zoe Kuyken, whom I love more than life itself; and Alison Yiangou for cultivating the ideas so they could express themselves fully, and for welcoming me into the Puckham Guesthouse, where much of the work was done. The book is immeasurably better because of conversations with and feedback from my daughters, my sister Ineke Kuyken, and many colleagues and friends: Angelique Augereau, Stephen Blumenthal, Tim Chiari, Rebecca Crane, Chris Cullen, Tim Dalgleish, Barney Dunn, Susan Earl, Gill Johnson, Tyson Joseph, Liz Lord, Shannon Maloney, Rachel Mariner, Jesús Montero-Marin, Ee-Lin Ong, Emmanuelle Peters, Malgosia Stepnik, Uta Tiggesmeir, Marc van Heyningen, Andreas Volstad, Erin Walker, and Shula Wolfenden. My colleague Yasmijn Slaghekke provided excellent editorial support in the final stages.

At The Guilford Press, Kitty Moore suggested the idea of this book and introduced me to Chris Benton. This book is infinitely better through Chris's skillful editing. She worked like a sculptor hewing the stone to reveal what it needed to be. They both believed in the book and in me, never stopped believing, and like the very best of friends held me to account at every stage in ways that improved the book.

Other books with The Guilford Press include *Mindfulness: Ancient Wisdom Meets Modern Psychology*, written with my friend and colleague Christina Feldman, and *Collaborative Case Conceptualization*, cowritten with my wonderful colleagues Christine Padesky and Robert Dudley. A forthcoming book, cowritten with my colleagues Paul Bernard and Ruth Baer, is a guide for mindfulness teachers, enabling them to introduce and teach the Mindfulness for Life curriculum. Thank you to my agent, Joelle Delbourgo.

There are leaders in the field of mindfulness whose friendship and support I have been privileged to have, among them Jon Kabat-Zinn for his tireless work to formulate how mindfulness can best serve in the mainstream of the contemporary world and his unwavering friendship and support. I also owe a debt of gratitude to Zindel Segal, Mark Williams, and John Teasdale, who developed mindfulness-based cognitive therapy and generously allowed me to explore how best to develop the curriculum's DNA so as make it as broadly accessible as possible. I am appreciative of the excellent teachers, trainers, and staff at the Oxford Mindfulness Foundation who continue to support the dissemination and evolution of this work: Merran Barber, Jo Cromarty, Sheila Gill, Sharon Hadley, Debbie Hu, Claire Kelly, Andy Phee, Jem Shackleford, Tim Sweeney, Andrew Waterhouse, Peter Yiangou, and many others. I am grateful as well to the people who attended our classes, with curiosity, openness, courage, trust, and patience, alongside a willingness to learn and use these ideas in their lives. Together we're developing a shared vision where these ideas help people to meet the challenges not only in their lives, but also in the wider world.

All my best work has been collaborative. My collaborators and mentors have included Ruth Baer, Aaron T. Beck, Paul Bernard, Sarah-Jayne Blakemore, Jud Brewer, Chris Brewin, Sarah Byford, Richard Byng, John Campbell, Rebecca Crane, Chris Cullen, Tim Dalgleish, Chris Dickens, Rob Dudley, Barney Dunn, Alison Evans, Christina Feldman, Tamsin Ford, Mark Greenberg, Rick Hecht, Felicia Huppert, Anke Karl, David Kessler, Tony Lavender, Glyn Lewis, Eric Loucks, Jesús Montero-Marin, Christine Padesky, Dave Richards, Jo Rycroft-Malone, Zindel Segal, Ilina Singh, Anne Speckens, Clara Strauss, Rod Taylor, John Teasdale, Obi Ukoumunne, Anne Maj van der Velden, Ed Watkins, Katherine Weare, Nicola Wiles, Jenny Wilks, Mark Williams, Alison Yiangou, and two research consortia, the WHOQOL Group and the MYRIAD Group. My research team has included Matt Allwood, Louise Aukland, Jennifer Baker-Jones, Corinna Baum, Shadi Beshai, Daniel Brett, Clare Bootle, Jess Cardy, Triona Casey, Aaron Causley, Eleanor-Rose Corney, Suzanne Cowderoy, Catherine Crane, Nicola Dalrymple, Kath de Wilde, Katie Fletcher, Claire Fothergill, Nora Goerg, Felix Gradinger, Rachel Hayes, Nils

Kappelmann, Maria Kempnich, Liz Lord, Jo MacKenzie, Karen Mansfield, Pete Mason, Emma Meldicot, Elizabeth Nuthall, Lucy Palmer, Ariane Petit, Alice Phillips, Isobel Pryor, Lucy Radl, Anam Raja, Jem Shackelford, Pooja Shah, Cara Simmance, Yasmijn Slaghekke, Anna Sonley, Holly Sugg, Harry Sutton, Laura Taylor, Alice Tickell, Kate Tudor, Rachael Vicary, Lucy Warriner, Kat White, Stephanie Wilde, and Matt Williams. My postgraduate students have included Anna Abel, Mark Allen, Modi Alsubaie, Chantal Baillie, Lisa Baxter, Andrew Bromley, Rachael Carrick, Colin Greaves, Emma Griffiths, Jenny Gu, J. J. Hill, Verena Hinze, Emily Holden, Vivienne Hopkins, Hans Kirschner, Kat Legge, Shannon Maloney, Jo Mann, Nicola Motton, Meyrem Musa, Kearnan Myall, Selina Nath, Dimitrious Tsivrikos, Anne Maj van der Velden, Andreas Volstad, and Alice Weaver.

My research has been supported by the National Institute for Health Research, the Wellcome Trust, the Sir John Ritblat Family Foundation, the Oxford Mindfulness Foundation, the Medical Research Council, and the University of Oxford.

As Einstein noted, we need a different way of thinking from that which created the challenges we're facing. We need a way of using the best science and ideas, wherever they come from, to be innovative and rigorous in finding meaningful, tractable and sustainable solutions. I don't claim to have written an original treatise. The last 50 years have seen some ideas and practices from contemplative traditions, psychology, and other disciplines become mainstream. Increasingly, the entangled nature of these ideas and the truth they are trying to represent are also being explored in creative and innovative ways. I would like to acknowledge my gratitude to some of the people whose ideas have most inspired me: Aaron T. Beck, Tara Brach, Barbara Fredrickson, Joseph Goldstein, Thich Nhat Hanh, Daniel Kahneman, Jack Kornfeld, and Ian McGilchrist. And they too of course drew on other traditions, ancient and modern, in religion, philosophy, the humanities, and psychology. Finally, I have drawn on David Treleaven's work to ensure these ideas and practices are offered with sensitivity to people with a history of trauma.

I apologize if I inadvertently neglected anyone I should have thanked or mentioned.

Introduction

A Life Well Lived:
Beginning with the End in Mind

Hiking in the Lake District of England, I stopped for lunch in a cemetery. There was a headstone with a name and this simple inscription: "A Life Well Lived." What does a life well lived look like? It's a question that we've all asked in one form or another. It's a question that has been asked for millennia by artists, from musicians to painters, dancers, sculptors, poets, and rappers, as well as philosophers and contemplatives.

An average life, around the world as of 2020, lasts 72 years, 4,000 weeks, or 26,000 days. As I write this, more than likely I've lived the balance of my days. How many years, weeks, and days have you lived of your life? And what does a life lived well look like for you? When I have asked people this question, here are some of the most typical responses:

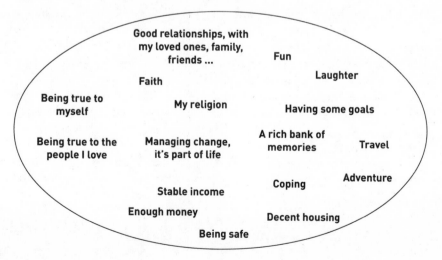

Good relationships, with my loved ones, family, friends ...

Fun

Faith

Laughter

Being true to myself

My religion

Having some goals

Being true to the people I love

Managing change, it's part of life

A rich bank of memories

Travel

Stable income

Coping

Adventure

Enough money

Decent housing

Being safe

Of course, everyone is different, and everyone will have a different list. What we value also changes at different stages of life. I'd like to suggest that a life well lived means living with a sense of direction and purpose, accompanied by good friends, awake to all of life's myriad and varied moments, equipped to cope with the inevitable ups and downs of life.

Is This Book for You?

If you're interested in living your life well, this book is for you. You may have a nagging feeling that your life isn't quite as you'd imagined. Or maybe you appreciate that you have a good life—and you'd like to keep it that way or even build on these foundations, because who knows what the years ahead may bring. But what does mindfulness have to do with this?

Mindfulness: Three Keys to Living Well

Mindfulness offers three keys that can help you unlock a life well lived. This book gives you access to them no matter how familiar you are with mindfulness. Perhaps you've been intrigued by the term, or taken a course, or practiced mindfulness for a while but let it lapse, as so many of us do. This book offers you a way to keep the three keys to hand for life.

Key 1: Befriending Your Mind

"My mind can be my worst enemy or best friend," said Raheem Sterling, a young English soccer player. Sterling is known for inspiring others through his work ethic, for his family values, and for raising awareness of important social issues. He meditates because it helps him befriend his mind, which in turn helps him with his sport, mental health, and wider work.

What does friendship mean to you? What words or phrases best describe your friendships? What does a good friend do for you—now and over years, through the good and the bad patches of your life?

> Mindfulness is about our mind being and becoming our best friend.

I've posed these questions to hundreds of people in workshops around the world, and here is what people said most often:

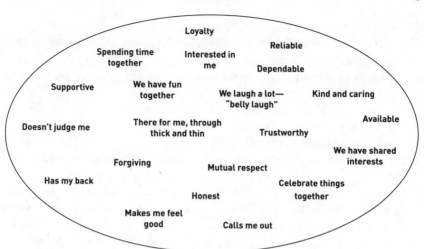

Does your idea of a good friend describe how you feel about your own mind? Maybe you already talk to yourself in affirming ways, with messages like "You've got this," "Steady," "Take a breath," "I've got your back; it will be okay." Or maybe the voice you use with yourself is critical—"I can't do that"—or demanding: "I don't have time." If you already have a sense of your mind as a friend, this book will help you develop that friendship further. You can choose to befriend your mind so that it becomes as practiced and natural as putting on your shoes before you go out. If you don't feel like your mind is your friend, you'll learn in the following pages how to change that, whatever challenges it throws up and amid whatever life circumstances you're in.

Key 2: Using Your Values as Your Compass

Certain ideas and values have become mainstream:

- I measure myself by how much I get done, what I'm bringing in, whether it's on a personal level or for the greater good, sort of like my "Gross Domestic Product."
- I put myself first because it is a dog-eat-dog world.
- I've got to always be on point—you know, look amazing, stay youthful, stay in shape, be attractive, and show that I'm making it in life.
- If I let my guard down, I'll get taken advantage of.
- Busyness is good.

- Being tough is good; being kind is soft.
- Being in the spotlight, that's what gives my life meaning. I'm *this close* to striking it rich, if only I can score the perfect job, hit that jackpot, blow up as an influencer, or just start hanging with the right crowd.

From an early age, we feel pressure to have an opinion—about who we are, other people, what we like and don't like, our favorite this or that, what we want to do when we grow up. We may claim certain "values" just to avoid uncertainty or to avoid feeling ashamed of not knowing what our values are. With all the pressure on us to do well, be better, achieve, prove we deserve our place in the world, or look a certain way, we may simply adopt prevalent ideas without question. When we do, we may end up pursuing someone else's vision for our life. Of course productivity is necessary, but few people at the end of their lives look back and say, "I had a good life because I was productive and successful in this dog-eat-dog, getting-ahead world." And if they do, did it make them and the people around them happy? Ask yourself right now what makes *you* happy. What or whom do you care most about? What are you passionate about? No need to overthink, just note what comes up, then let it go and see what else comes up. And don't worry if not much arises; that's fine too.

Your answers to these questions of what matters most point to your values. We're all different, and an important part of living well is knowing what's meaningful to us.

Here are some of the values that people often mention.

Values are at the root of mindfulness; they guide how we are in the world and what we say and do. And just as important, they guide what we don't say or do. If family is a foundational value, this shapes choices and even lives. Faith provides a sense of belonging and meaning. Everyone's story involves learning a set of values. My father had a strong work and family ethic, developed in very difficult circumstances when he found himself the "man of the family" as a young boy interned in a concentration camp with his mother and younger sisters and brother. Throughout his life he provided selflessly for his family through hard work. I know he regarded the savings he left behind to provide for my mother and my sisters and me a key part of his life work.

This book will bring to life how your values can be your sense of direction, your compass, the route map on your phone. In the pages ahead you'll explore your values and how they can guide you. I'll encourage you to embrace your values and to be courageous enough to value what is truly important. The

> Wherever you are, whatever you're doing, your values, like a compass, point you in the right direction.

landscape of our lives, our family, our school, workplace, community, planet is created by human minds and hearts. It can be tempting to retreat to routine, to where we feel safe, to what we know. But try asking, "Is this enlarging and in line with my values or reassuring but ultimately diminishing?" Enlarge your mind, your relationships, your life, your sense of what is possible in the world. Seek out what enlarges you, whatever that is. It may be people in your life, sports, art, a favorite phrase, or an idea. Who and what enlarges you? Can they be what protects you, vitalizes you, and gives you a sense of purpose?

Key 3: Waking Up and Paying Attention

There are a lot of pulls on our attention, and this can give us a sense of being fragmented. With all the demands on us, it's easy to react by checking out and sleepwalking through life. Zoning out can be comfortable, but there are many good reasons to live with a sense of being fully awake.

Attention is one of your most important resources. What you focus on shapes what you think, your decisions, what you feel, and ultimately, your reality. It's like the spotlight that illuminates certain conversations, people, successes, problems, feelings, while leaving others

> Leading the life we want means waking up and paying attention.

in the shadows. How much of today have you been awake? I don't mean awake literally; I mean awake in the sense of feeling alive. Twenty-five percent, 50 percent, most of the day? In the pages ahead you'll find ways you can learn to pay attention to how you spend your days—and the moments of each day. Every moment is already here, waiting for you to pay attention to it. In a sense you don't need to do anything differently. It is more of an adjustment in *how you approach your day*, choosing to pay attention, on purpose, with attitudes of curiosity and friendliness.

When you're guided by your values, you befriend your mind, and you live with awareness, you focus on what matters, and your deepest values and daily life come together in a way that feels whole. Vulnerability can align with strength, kindness can be a force for positive change, compassion can be tough, and love can seep into and out from the people in your life.

Developing Mindfulness—through Practice and through Life

You can make friends with your mind, figure out what truly matters to you, and reclaim your focus by practicing mindfulness. When you wake up and stay aware, you can develop these qualities and skills in your everyday life. In time life itself becomes the mindfulness practice.

Although many people associate mindfulness with meditation, in this book we use the term "mindfulness practice" because of the importance of the word *practice*. You're practicing so you can apply the three keys to living well in your daily life. Each chapter in this book presents mindfulness practices, each with a specific purpose and approach. Some help you discover what's important to you, some help you maintain focus, some foster qualities like kindness, and some lead to deeper understanding. But mindfulness can also be integrated into your life by changing how you approach your regular activities, and that is also a big part of each chapter in the book.

What might mindfulness practice look like in your life? Like everything else, it will evolve over time, and I invite you to discover what mindfulness for life can mean for you. No doubt you know that most things that are worthwhile take effort and time. This is certainly true of cultivating our minds and bodies. And when you see mindfulness practice as a way to renew and replenish yourself, rather than something you should do, it becomes something you genuinely want or even need to do.

Questions and Obstacles:
An Integral Part of Learning Mindfulness

Inevitably, obstacles and questions arise when you practice mindfulness for life. These are not only to be expected but can teach us something. Of course this doesn't make the journey easy; it means acknowledging difficult stuff we may have been pushing away and reveals the disconnect between how we'd like our lives to be and how they are. But by staying aware of this gap, with interest and care, we can begin to explore where we are and what path it is pointing us to.

Each chapter will name the common questions and obstacles and help you with responses. You will meet two guides that are there to help throughout the book: the Ancient Oak, who has a deep and wide knowledge that draws on contemplative traditions, philosophy, the humanities, and the arts; and the Barefoot Professor, who knows a lot about psychology but also has a passable knowledge of other mainstream science. These characters don't take themselves too seriously—not because what they're saying isn't important, but because they know that the more you know, the more you realize that things are complicated and there is still so much to learn.

> ### The Ancient Oak: Obstacles as Teachers
>
> There is a story of a monastery where there was one monk who coughed during the meditation, snored at night, and broke wind without compunction. The other monks complained to the abbot, "He's ruining our meditation, makes it hard to sleep at night, and stinks the place out. Can you please do something about him?" The abbot smiled and responded, "I pay that monk to be here; his coughing, snoring, and flatulence are all intended to help you develop your patience, equanimity, and kindness."

Can Mindfulness Practice Really Help You Live Well?

Over many years, skepticism about mindfulness has been prevalent. One of the most common myths about it is that it's something we must do—another major task to undertake. After doing some mindfulness training, many people say, "I did it for a while, but then I stopped"—because it was too hard, it didn't pay off in big ways, they didn't have time, it didn't seem to fit with their modern lifestyle. But what is "it," and what does it mean not to be able to "do it?" Every skill we've discussed—awareness, paying attention, learning—is an innate human resource. It is simply impossible to stop doing "it." I'd like to suggest a different way of thinking about mindfulness. If we don't go to the gym, we lose our strength; if we don't work out, we lose our fitness. While this analogy is often used for mindfulness practice, you can't unlearn something that is natural or unknow something you've learned deeply. Mindfulness training is simply revealing and cultivating natural human qualities. Is it worth the effort to continue practicing? Only you can decide.

Of course, mindfulness isn't for everyone. And we all resist change, at least at first. Hedonistic pleasure is nice. Waking sleep is seductive; it means we don't have to face up to all sorts of realities and challenges. Fear is a powerful emotion. How we deal with these obstacles to practicing mindfulness for life will be addressed throughout the book, with each chapter troubleshooting the most common issues as they come up.

With practice, I hope you'll see why mindfulness is becoming mainstream: it can help us live well in the contemporary world. It is an antidote to busyness and distractedness, however compelling these can be. Many mindfulness practices have been used by people for thousands of years. The science of mindfulness is coming of age. This confluence of ancient and modern is what gives it depth and realism. Mindfulness can be masculine and feminine, it can move in and retreat, it is strong and vulnerable, ordinary and profound, eminently practical and potentially transformative. Mindfulness skills have extraordinary potential to help us respond to some of the challenges we're facing in today's world. It can help us understand how we react and behave. It can help us respond with greater wisdom and compassion.

> Mindfulness is not a magic fix. It requires a sense of curiosity, realistic expectations, an ongoing commitment, and discipline.

When I say "us," I mean us as individuals, but also as communities and as wider humanity. But for this potential to be realized we need it to be taught and learned well, applied with care and always with solid foundational values.

I hope that you will integrate the ideas and practices into your life, rather than viewing them as a temporary Band-Aid or a sort of optional hobby. Like the commitment of a lifelong friendship, we don't make it lightly. We make it because the friendship is important to us, we know it will require hard work and we'll sometimes neglect it.

To help you integrate mindfulness into your life, it helps to ask questions like:

- What, or rather how, do I want to be? Busy, jangled, compulsive . . . ?
- Why should I make this commitment? What value might mindfulness add to my life?
- How can I integrate mindfulness into my life, so it is relevant and helps me?
- How can I stay motivated to use these ideas and mindfulness practices in my busy life?
- How can my mindfulness practice evolve through the different stages of life, as my needs and responsibilities shift and change?

The Ancient Oak and the Barefoot Professor: Living a Good Life

The Ancient Oak: Aristotle thought that a life well lived means character (*ēthikós*), purpose (*telos*), and virtue (*arete*). These three together create a sense of contentment, meaning, and well-being (*eudaimonia*). What is helpful about this? First, Aristotle is saying that well-being is something much deeper and enduring than happiness. And second, living well is something we can become good at. There are lots of ways these ideas have been developed. Ilina Singh, a professor at the University of Oxford, has suggested that a good life includes not just an individual, but also the groups of people and the wider world the person is part of.

The Barefoot Professor: Often we think money, having pleasant experiences, and avoiding pain are what make us happy. And of course, laughter, good food, buying or having nice things, excitement, entertainment, physical intimacy, beautiful things. These all make us feel good, but usually only for as long as we have them (this is sometimes called hedonic pleasure), or we're always striving for more, better (this is sometimes called the hedonic treadmill). Psychology has shown that we get in the way of our own happiness through our tendency to want more, to judge what we have against what others have, or what we feel we should have. This makes hedonic pleasure quite fragile compared to the more enduring contentment Aristotle and wider well-being Ilina Singh are pointing us to. Psychology may be a lot younger than ancient wisdom, but it has yielded some scientific studies showing how mindfulness can support well-being in different groups of people and settings—and when it doesn't.

This book will show you how you can learn to become aware in ways that help you live well. It will help you wake up, pay attention, get to know your body and mind, learn to appreciate the good things, while also dealing with stress, problems, losses, and pain. You'll discover how to gain a fresh perspective, be kind to yourself, know when to accept things, and when to make changes. All of this will help you take care of yourself and others with wisdom, courage, and openness to learning.

Mindfulness in Real Life—*for* Life

Throughout our lives, we encounter significant milestones such as starting school, going through puberty, leaving home, beginning work, forming and ending relationships, switching jobs, retiring, and dealing with changes in our health. What you'll learn can help you stay attuned to your evolving aspirations, values, and beliefs, and the new directions you want to take during the various stages of life. Inevitably we'll face unexpected challenges: losing a job, relationships breaking down, ill health, people dying, our own inevitable decline and death. We have the capacity to show extraordinary resilience in the face of these challenges, as is plain to see if we look at our personal and collective history. Think back on some of the changes you've weathered. Even in the last hundred years, collectively we've weathered world wars, changes in the world's demography, economic booms and downturns, and pandemics like Covid-19. I want this book to help you on a lifelong journey of learning mindfulness, from first being introduced to mindfulness, through integrating it into to your life, through going further and deeper with the development of awareness, understanding, and compassion.

Bringing Mindfulness to Life: Sam, Mohammed, Ling, and Sophia

Over the years I've learned so much from my teachers and mentors, people who participated in my classes and workshops, and colleagues, as well as in my life more generally. Out of these experiences I've created four people, composites of individuals I've met, to show how mindfulness can take shape in real life. They have the job of illustrating not just what can be learned, what's new, interesting, and joyful, but importantly all the problems or issues that require troubleshooting along the way.

Sam is a nurse in his 20s, training as an ICU specialist nurse practitioner, who was drifting through his life until he reset with a few simple realizations.

> SAM: *My job is more than just work to me, I'm seriously passionate about it. And honestly, I'm not complicated—hitting the pedals, and gaming, love it. Just like how I keep my bike in check with a weekly tune-up, I've gotta do the same for myself, making sure I eat right and catch up on sleep when I go a bit too hard.*

If, as for Sam, mindfulness helps us tune in to what is good in our life, and feel better, we get curious and want to learn more.

Mohammed is in his 30s, a former athlete, father, husband, now a full-time homemaker—his faith is foundational in his life. To live well, he had to learn to live with chronic pain, the legacy of an injury that ended his athletic aspirations.

Ling is in her 40s, divorced, a single mother to teenage kids, juggling to keep all the balls in her full life up in the air, working a job she doesn't like much.

LING: *You know, I never really picked up swimming when I was a kid. So, when I first got introduced to mindfulness, it kinda felt like someone was trying to nudge me into diving into my friend's most-loved swimming hole. I had this vivid image of standing on the brink, testing the waters of mindfulness—all the excuses I had for just turning back and not giving it a shot. But you know what? I took that first step, "dipped my toes" into it. And after that? Honestly, it's been quite different from what I thought.*

Waking up was not easy or painless for Ling, and she realized she needed to make changes to her life.

Sophia is a retired teacher, mother, grandmother. Retirement was a major transition for her.

SOPHIA: *I feel like I have been granted two lives, the first, and the second when I woke up and realized I only have one life!*

These four characters have, in their own way, first been introduced to mindfulness, then integrated it into their lives, and then made a commitment to taking it further so it is a lifelong process. My hope is they will inspire you to integrate these ideas into your life in the same ways.

Twelve Stepping Stones to Mindfulness for Life

This book contains twelve chapters that you can think of as a series of stepping stones. Early stepping stones are about inhabiting your body, vulnerable and resilient, constant, and ever changing, life seeking and ultimately mortal. Your body and mind are united; joy or suffering in one reverberates in the other.

Later stepping stones are about how you can keep a sense of perspective and balance and live as best you can with the inevitable changes and challenges in your life.

You can visit each chapter again and again, so you learn more about the ways you can integrate all that you're learning that will be helpful in your life. In this sense the idea of stepping stones becomes more like a set of skills you can use in different ways at different times, throughout your life.

Being the Change You'd Like to See in the World

Mahatma Gandhi suggested that the best way to change the world is by *being* the change we want to see in the world. We've started with the end in mind, so you can glimpse where we're headed and the path you're walking. We'll return to the idea of being the change you want to see in the world again and again. And in the last chapter of this book we'll take stock. As you go along, you'll have to see for yourself if this is true for you. A friend alongside you might say, "Laugh along the way, have fun, be brave, accept the missteps, maybe even learn from them, celebrate the successes—we're in this together and I've got your back."

1

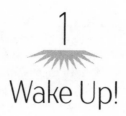

Wake Up!

"I am sleepwalking through life. I want my mojo back."

"My life feels like a long to-do-list. I feel overwhelmed a lot of the time."

"My father worked so hard all his life, always making plans for his retirement. Then he died of a brain tumor at age 62. He missed out on so much—I don't want to make that mistake."

We can all sleepwalk through our days, checking off all the things we have to do and tuning out when it all gets to be too much. This can become a habit—how we live our lives. How much of the time do you operate like this? When does it serve you? When does it not? And at what cost?

> LING: *I drove home my usual route, running late as usual. As I pulled up onto the drive, I realized that, for most of my commute, I'd been totally lost in thought. So, what was I thinking about? Busy, busy. I remembered the case I'd heard in court that day, I worried about everything I need to do tomorrow, I planned what I could cook for dinner given that the fridge was empty, I glanced at my phone and saw loads of notifications. I turned on the radio because I didn't want to think about it anymore.*

Ling's life is full—her work, solo parenting two teenagers, running a house—and it can be relentless.

Modern airplanes can fly on autopilot or have the pilot take control. Airline pilots can choose to turn on a plane's autopilot so the plane flies itself. This enables the pilot to consult the instruments and maps or take a break. The autopilot can even do some things better than pilots because it follows programmed

> How can you move from endlessly working through the have-to-dos of life to being more like a human being and less like a human doing?

algorithms that aren't prone to human error. But sometimes the pilot is needed because his or her judgment is better than autopilot. Our minds are a bit the same. There are many routine activities, Ling's commute to work for example, that can be done on autopilot. Many of these skills are incredibly complex, yet you can get on with them effectively in the background. For example, you're reading this without having to spell out every letter and word; you've learned to read and make sense of what is being said automatically and rapidly. Your breathing, heartbeat, balance, posture, and so many other functions are also being managed on autopilot. Some are deep in our nature, such as our breathing. Others you've learned to do growing up, so you don't have to think about them in the normal run of life.

There is so much going on in the background of your mind and body all the time that you're not aware of. This is a good thing—it means those essential tasks are getting done. And it allows you to choose to turn your attention to other things—new things you're learning for the first time, something you're choosing to focus on, something that urgently needs your attention, a conversation. Autopilot frees you up to attend to what you choose to focus on, while essential functions take place in the background—breathing, balancing, digesting, checking your surroundings to make sure you're safe.

As for a pilot, autopilot is there when you need it. Like a pilot, you can choose to activate it or deactivate it. What does this look like in everyday life?

MOHAMMED: *I always walk the kids to school, and it's usually a pretty stressful routine—get them up, fed, out the door and to school on time. But today was a little bit different. Even though we had spilled breakfast cereal and lost homework, we set out earlier than normal because the kids wanted to. They wanted to check out the spider webs on the way and to pick up chestnuts underneath the big chestnut tree. We had time, which meant that we stopped to actually see the intricate spider's web and choose the best chestnuts. As we got close to the school, my kids started pointing and waving excitedly at a fully packed double-decker bus driving by; quite a few of the passengers were looking out the windows. Ah, now I got it; my kids were waving at a kid they knew well sitting at the front of the top deck. But then several people on the bus waved back, thinking my kids were waving at them—we laughed, strangers waving at each other on their morning commute. I smiled, actually really smiled, as if the morning was unfolding in slow motion and technicolor.*

What we'll explore in this chapter is what it means to wake up and live with a sense of purpose, joy, and ease. Mohammed's example of taking a bit more time for the school run illustrates how this created small moments of appreciation and laughter. We always wake up in the morning from our night's sleep, but what I mean here is properly waking up. We'll start where we are, with all that makes up our days.

Waking Up to Our Everyday Lives

How we spend our days is, of course, how we spend our lives.
—ANNIE DILLARD

This is such a simple and powerful idea. If you're to lead the life you want, that means paying attention to how you spend your days—and the moments that make up each day. It's also very good news; our everyday life is already here waiting for us to pay attention to it. In a sense you don't need to do anything new. Mindfulness of everyday activities is simply making an adjustment in *how you approach your day*, choosing to pay attention, on purpose, *with an attitude of interest and care.*

The Ancient Oak and the Barefoot Professor: Curiosity

The Ancient Oak: Contemplative traditions encourage us to be focused and disciplined, so that we can see things more clearly and learn from our experience. The best teachers encourage their students not to take what they say on faith, but rather examine everything for themselves: "The wise test the purity of gold by burning, cutting and examining it by means of a piece of touchstone." (These words are attributed to the Buddha in the Discourses of the Buddha.) That is to say, they check it out for themselves.

The Barefoot Professor: This reminds me of Einstein saying, "It is the supreme art of the teacher to awaken joy in creative expression and knowledge." He was pointing to learning for yourself how to be interested in your experiences, small and large, the everyday and the profound, and asking, "What can I learn?" More than this, learning with a sense of joy.

Eating Mindfully—Small Fruit, Big Message

An everyday activity we all do, and which many of us do on autopilot much of the time, is eating. When infants and toddlers encounter something for the first time, they bring to it a sense of awe and wonder, what's sometimes called "beginner's mind." *Beginner's mind* means recapturing this sense of seeing things as if for the first time.

SOPHIA: *One weekend I was taking care of my grandson, Noah. I had bought some fresh strawberries at the market earlier in the day because I knew Noah had recently started to eat solid foods. It was time to introduce him to strawberries, so I handed him one in his high chair. He squashed it in his hands, with delight at its softness and the way, as he crushed it, it changed into mush. Then he put his hands and the strawberry mush to his mouth. His eyes lit up, and his whole face creased with the sweetness of the strawberry first on his lips and then, when he realized he really liked it, in his mouth. In that moment he looked like he'd discovered something amazing, which he had, the feel and taste of a fresh strawberry. I gave him a second strawberry and had an idea. It was just the two of us, and I thought, to hell with it; no one is watching, I am going to eat this strawberry exactly like Noah, mirroring what he does, move by move. Oh my, we both enjoyed the feel, smell, and taste of the fresh strawberries—and we laughed, belly laughed. It was messy—I couldn't get away with this in a restaurant—but it was fun. Noah has beginner's mind because he is an infant who has never tasted a strawberry.*

Sophia is bringing beginner's mind to eating a strawberry. There is an expression, "coming to our senses." Sophia is quite literally coming to her senses by bringing curiosity to the fullness and richness of the strawberry, not assuming how the strawberry will feel, smell, and taste. We can all do this. We can put a strawberry in our mouth with an expectation of how it will be and not actually pause and smell and taste how it is in this moment. Nowadays there are many types of strawberries—they all taste and feel a bit different. I discovered wild strawberries in an overgrown churchyard recently and tried one. Its taste was interesting, textured, not at all sweet. It tasted like a strawberry but not like any strawberry I had ever eaten. This can be true of how we choose to meet our day, our life. When we do, a whole world of detail, color, and richness reveals itself.

Yes, habit is essential, but sometimes what we've automated is not the background, same-old, same-old—it is our lives. There are also many moments in the day that we perhaps write off as "dead space" or part of what makes us feel our day is full or busy: getting dressed, brushing our hair, commuting, dropping kids off at school, waiting for a bus or train to arrive, riding an elevator. But are these moments dead space? Or are they moments when you can come to your senses and ask, "How am I doing right now? How is my mind [calm or agitated, for example]? How is my body [energized or tired]?" These moments are moments in which you can check in and then move on with your day with a greater sense of purpose and connection.

Mindfulness of Everyday Activities

Consider all the everyday things you do throughout the day—washing your hands, walking from place to place, attending to the notifications on your cell phone, getting a message from someone you haven't heard from for a while, talking to people, the moment you wake up, the moments before you fall asleep, eating a strawberry, the moment someone shows you a kindness, a cherry tree in blossom, greeting someone you care about who you haven't seen for a while, the first cup of coffee or tea of the day, really being with a friend, and so on.

Each of these things provides an opportunity to pay attention, to come to your senses. Can you make this intentional and be curious? For example, as you wash your hands, can you come back to the direct experience of the water, soap, and your hands moving across each other? As you drink a cup of coffee or tea, can you really taste, smell, and savor it?

Throughout the day, lift and broaden your gaze. What do you see? Are there things you're missing because you're either not looking or you've made up your mind very quickly about what is there? Can you see it with begin-

> It is a simple but powerful idea—choosing *how and what you pay attention to.*

ner's mind? What is it like to do something that you normally do on autopilot with beginner's mind? When you pay attention, you add depth and vibrancy to whatever you're paying attention to. Now consider *what you're choosing to pay attention to.* How would it be to choose to notice the good moments within a day? If you can be more fully present to these moments in your day, you can more fully experience the joy, beauty, love, pleasures, and rewards of your life.

PRACTICE: Ten-Finger Appreciation

You can follow along on our website.

Our lives contain many things that are good, beautiful, lovely. This practice involves intentionally bringing attention to some of the many blessings in our lives that you usually overlook.

Begin by finding a comfortable position and take a moment to connect with your body. Then take hold of the thumb of one hand with the other hand, feeling the contact of skin on skin.

And now bring to mind an object in your home that you appreciate and feel the sense of appreciation that you have for this object.

Now let go of that object in your mind and your thumb and take hold of your index finger and bring to mind something in nature that you appreciate, feeling the sense of appreciation and gratitude, tuning in to sensations.

Continue in this way, letting go of your index finger and taking hold of the next finger and bringing to mind something you appreciate about a person that you know. Keep going with specific things for which you feel a sense of appreciation until you've worked through all ten fingers of your hands.

MOHAMMED: *My son's smile when he kicked the football through my legs into the goal. I loved that.*

SOPHIA: *The fall colors of the tree in front of my house when I came home yesterday afternoon.*

The reason I suggest using all ten fingers is to really broaden your horizon to as wide a range of instances as possible. It helps to really explore all the small moments of the day that can be appreciated, moments that may be overlooked because they're dismissed as trivial.

> SAM: *My go-to travel coffee cup that I take to work. It's like my little slice of home that I bring to work. Plus I just love good coffee, and the coffee they serve in the hospital is undrinkable. My coffee makes the workday a whole lot better.*

Sam smiled as he relayed this example. The smile is important, because it is his body expressing joy. You can learn to notice and allow these positive states and expressions, even celebrate them. Creating a list in your head is a good start, but this is not a tick-box exercise and definitely not a think-positive exercise. Positive thinking is the opposite of paying attention to how things are, and it can easily backfire. You can easily wind up feeling like you fall short. Instead, appreciation is a simple, light noticing of good, small moments in your day and really opening up to these and allowing yourself to enjoy them. It's a *practice*—something to do with your mind *and your body*. See if you can start by noticing what it feels like in your body when you bring these instances to mind. When you do this, what do you learn? More than likely, you'll see how these can become a mini reliving of good experiences—if you stay with it, you can have a sense of really taking in the good.

TROUBLESHOOTING: Common Early Obstacles

Here are some examples of the difficulties people run into as they first learn about mindfulness.

Maybe you're thinking, "Hokum, that's just not for me." Or "So what? I notice things. Now what?" I've had these thoughts myself. As the Ancient Oak and the Barefoot Professor said, don't take anyone's word for it; try it for yourself. All I do ask is, as best you can, approach them with a sense of curiosity and open-mindedness. Be patient. Adopt a sense of "Who knows what I might learn?" It's a bit like gardening. When you plant a seed or small plant, you have to give it time to grow, bed in, and mature. The rest of the book is about this cultivation.

Wake up to what? I don't get it. Well, that is the discovery, and it will likely include both difficulties and delights, in both our lives and the wider world.

> ### The Ancient Oak
>
> The origin of the word *concentration* in Greek is *kentron*, a sharp point in the center or the verb *to prick*. Our concentration literally pricks us awake.

LING: *I work as a court reporter. I'm just transcribing what's said in court, but that doesn't mean I don't take it in. I hear some terrible things, assaults, sexual violence, people cheating each other. Some of the child custody cases are heart wrenching. I'd be lying if I said it didn't affect me—it does.*

It's easy to understand why Ling might choose, or even need, to tune out at work. But as we'll see in the chapters ahead, while not easy, waking up helped her make important changes.

Whoa, this is all way too much, too fast. As with anything new— exercising, a new job, a new relationship—it's wise to take small steps. Trust yourself as you go along, taking small steps that give you a chance to notice what is and isn't okay, alert you to any red flags, where the boundaries are, and guide you away from trouble. If our lives are full, this may be the time to go easy on ourselves, not add more pressure.

LING: *My life is so full. I have so much on my plate, I'm often tired, and frankly often irritable; I don't have much space to do anything on top of juggling my life, let alone mindfulness. All this paying attention—frankly, I'd rather not. Often on a busy day, when my kids are acting out, I give myself a break, pour myself a drink, and watch TV. I am choosing to take some time out from the world.*

Our experience is created from moment to moment, one moment setting the context for the next. This is quite profound, and getting a sense of what this means and particularly what it means for our agency (what I do this morning in part determines my function and well-being later and tomorrow) requires some practice. Take your time. These ideas and practices are intended to be for life, *for life.* That is, they're designed to help you have a life well lived, throughout your life.

Mindfulness, meditation, or anything that involves sitting still and clearing my mind just makes me want to get up and do something more interesting or useful. This restlessness can be very pervasive and compelling. Trying to stay present can make the restlessness even stronger. Try acknowledging and naming it: "Ah, that's restlessness." See if there are any whispering voices driving it—"Get busy, keep moving." Can you get curious about restlessness—how strong is it, whether it comes and goes, and what it's like if you don't listen to the whispering voice's commands? What's it like when you do? Then, firmly and kindly reorient your attention, to somewhere in the body that is grounded and steady or something outside that can hold your attention.

I find it hard to see anything to appreciate, and even if I do, I can't really relate to it. Some people find appreciation difficult for all sorts of reasons.

SAM: *Summoning up ten things to savor felt like I was taking a pop quiz and failing big time. I had to cut myself some slack. It turns out finding a few gems is fine for now, even tiny ones like a coffee count too.*

LING: *For me pleasure in my body is a slow burn. Normally my body just feels stressed. But when something good happens, I can notice little flickers of change. They're subtle and take time to come out. If I rush to my body too quickly, it snuffs out those flickers. I learned to pay attention to my body only once positive juices are fully flowing—sorry I'm mixing metaphors—once the flickers have taken hold, and I can then notice them a bit more. I have learned it's best for me to start with thinking about the good stuff, and only when I am confident that there is something there to pay attention to do I turn to my body.*

Finally, many people have beliefs that dampen or even block pleasant experiences—"I don't deserve this," "This won't last," or "This isn't real." These are powerful thoughts. Recognizing them as thoughts gives us a chance to step back and see them as thoughts, not facts. The rest of the book, especially the chapters on appreciating the life you have (Chapter 4), befriending (Chapter 7), and responding wisely (Chapter 9), will help you notice and respond to these self-sabotaging thoughts.

Waking Up in Real Life, for Life

After the Ecstasy, the Laundry
—JACK KORNFIELD

This is one of the best book titles I know. What mindfulness teacher Jack Kornfield is saying is that when mindfulness practices offer us moments of insight, peace, and happiness—the ecstasy—this begs the question "What next?" The answer: the laundry! He means we might learn to enjoy and savor moments, even have whole days, when we feel at ease, but all the have-to-dos, challenges, and discomforts of life will still be there—the laundry. Can we bring an attitude of curiosity to the "laundry" as well as the "ecstasy"? And here's the kicker: that's not only okay; it's what we need to do to keep moving forward.

Do any of these statements ring true?

- Everyone's life seems more together than mine. Why can't I get my act together?
- I have this idea of what my life should be, but I'm in a job that's a far

cry from that idea. (This could apply equally to a relationship, where you live, etc.)

- I'm turning 18/21/30/40/50/60/70 this year. How did I get here? Why is my life not the way I imagined? I'll get my life together soon.

We can all feel like we're surviving rather than thriving. Like our lives are not quite as we'd like them to be. This can be in small, seemingly trivial moments. Perhaps lying in bed worrying about the day ahead or ruminating about something that happened during the day. Or they can be more significant events. For example, a tryout for a sports team, an application for college, an interview for a job, a child who needs to tell us something important, mentoring others, a romantic date, a birthday party, our wedding day, an anniversary. These moments, small and big, can also be overrun by habit—we do it the way we think we should or the way we've always done it. Someone put it like this: "a tyranny of should have, could have, would have." Or we're so full of worry, we're not actually present: "I hope it's going okay. I wonder if everyone's having a good time. Did I remember to . . . ?" When I got married, the best advice I got the day before my wedding day was "Enjoy it." I did. I enjoyed being with my wife, my friends, the food, the beautiful ceremony, the feeling of love that permeated the wedding, and the impromptu midnight swimming in the lake!

So how do you keep this sense of interest, joy, and vitality? How do you keep from slipping back into habit? How do you recapture your mojo? How do you live with a sense of purpose? You start by knowing where you're starting from.

PRACTICE: Pausing and Checking In

You can follow along on our website.

I'd like to invite you, *right now, in this moment*, to pause. Turn your attention inward to answer these questions:

What is the state of my mind right now? Is it alert or dull; curious or bored; vibrant or hazy . . . ? Try choosing a word or two to describe your mind in this moment.

What about your body? Scan through your body and see if there are any particular sensations. Any discomfort, ease, tightness, warmth, coolness? Can you describe your body in this moment, again with just a word or two?

See if you can welcome whatever you discover, like you'd welcome a guest into your home—whether it's something good, maybe a sense of curiosity, or something problematic, like a pain. You don't need to change or fix anything—your experience is already here. You're simply pausing and checking in. Just experiencing your mind and body in this moment, as they are, with an attitude of welcoming them like guests.

In this chapter I've been introducing the idea of waking up—why it's important and how to do it. In this exercise you've intentionally taken a pause and tuned in to what's happening in your mind and body. You've just taken the time to answer the question "How are you?" What's the honest answer? How are you?

Becoming more aware can help you live your life in ways that help you see things you hadn't seen before and in a way you don't normally see them. I want to describe now how you can take this idea further for a lifetime, so it becomes part of your life.

Getting the Day Off to a Good Start

It's time to start living the life you've imagined.
—HENRY JAMES

The way you start your day frames the whole day. If you can start the day well, you're more likely to be able to handle the inevitable issues the day throws up. Many ancient contemplative traditions suggest starting the day with some contemplation, prayer, or meditation. Starting our day with a sense of purpose and intention can become part of the fabric of our lives! Each day is a new day that you can choose to seize—*carpe diem*.

This short mindfulness practice offers a way to start the day by your taking a moment to reflect on the day ahead.

PRACTICE: Starting the Day

You can follow along on our website.

The start of the day can provide a number of points at which you can pause and really "wake up." It could be the moment you transition from sleep to wakefulness, or the moment just before or after you get out of bed, in the shower, exercising, as you eat some breakfast or commute to work. Everyone's day is different, but for most of us there are a few moments where you can pause and check in. Start by choosing a good moment where you can pause and think about the day ahead. In that moment . . .

Tune in to how you're doing, noting how your body is (rested or tired, for example) and how your mind is (alert or drowsy).

Now turn your attention to your breath and body, noticing the sensations of breathing in your belly or chest.

Riding the waves of a few breaths can steady you. You don't need to do anything about your breathing; mostly this happens automatically. That's why bringing your attention to the breath can be so helpful; it's something that's always there taking care of itself.

Now take a few moments to think about the day ahead. What are you looking forward to? What are you worried about? Are there any commitments you'd like to make to yourself about how you'd like the day to be? Pause to maybe make these commitments to yourself, perhaps being specific, saying to yourself, "Today I will . . ." or "I will move though my day with an attitude of curiosity. . . ." It's important to make this positive: "I will . . ." rather than "I won't. . . ." Try to see in your mind's eye how the day might pan out as you'd like it to.

Each day is a chance to start again, choosing how you want to be today.

When this practice becomes part of how you start your day, you can develop it further. It can be helpful to think about what is important to you, what is meaningful, what you value. This could be to be effective, laugh more, or be creative, have fun, be true to yourself, to be respectful of others, to contribute to things you care about, even take time to do nothing. What's important to you could be determination, security, to be a good father/mother/daughter/son/partner; to be kind, to be loving, to be honest, to have fun. Keep it simple and manageable. You can then revisit this intention during the day, dropping into moments when what you've committed to is actually happening. This is about clarifying what's important to you—your values—so you can live in ways more aligned with your values.

The Starting the Day practice is simple. Once you get the hang of it, it can be done in just a few minutes, as part of how you start your day, in the same way you learned to start your day with brushing your teeth. At the start of the day you choose to intentionally check in, come to your body and mind, and then set an intention for the day. Keep it real, specific, simple, and manageable. Frame it positively, as how you want your life to be. Then throughout the day you can check in to see how you're doing. In time it can even become a habit!

SAM: *I was doing an advanced practicum in the Intensive Care Unit of a general hospital. One day I roll in after a marathon shift, emotionally drained. What's my genius move? Fire up the computer game, of course. Friends online, bets flying, and before I know it, it's 3:00 A.M. No dinner, 50 bucks down, and I'm a wreck. I crash into bed, knowing the alarm's set for 7:00, and I'm back in the hospital at 8:00. I realized gaming's not doing me any favors.*

So I told myself, "Let's make a change. A small change is fine." I decided to kick off each day eating something, preferably something healthy. So next time I shopped I stocked up on decent cereals. Milk? Not always in my fridge. Enter cereal bars. It may sound small, but it means I am getting some food before my shift. I'll deal with the gaming later.

*The Barefoot Professor: Research Shows
That Everyday Mindfulness Can Improve Our Well-Being*

Studies have shown that how people approach their day impacts well-being. They typically use a method called *experience sampling*. This means asking thousands of people throughout their day how they are doing, what they are doing, and how they are approaching their day. This type of study can provide insights into the moment-by-moment dynamics of our lives and our experience, answering the question "What shapes well-being?"

What do I mean by "How people approach their day"?

Psychology studies consistently show that a particular way of approaching things, rumination, is associated with feeling worse. Rumination is where we try to figure out why we feel the way we do. Contrary to what we think, "If only I could figure out why I feel sad, then I could fix it," rumination rarely helps; mostly it makes us feel worse.

Another set of studies shows that approaching each moment with a sense of awareness can be more important than what we're actually doing (although of course that's important too). Being mindful, as a general rule, seems to be associated with well-being.

Finally, more recent studies are showing that bringing moments of mindfulness and appreciation to our day improves our well-being.

The implication of this research is that it can really pay off to try, as best you can, to approach your day with a sense of intentionality and awareness. Of course, your basic temperament and life circumstances are important, but how you relate to each moment and each day is something you can change. There is a growing body of research showing that these are skills that we can learn. Richie Davidson, a professor at the University of Wisconsin, has gone so far as to suggest that well-being is a skill we can learn through practice. That's quite radical

Ending the Day

The end of each day can be a time for taking stock. Instead of ending the day collapsing exhausted into bed like a heap or, worse, lying in bed ruminating about the day just gone and worrying about the day ahead, the end of the day can be a moment for reflection, appreciation, and then letting go. This mindfulness practice is a way to intentionally take a moment to review the day before you go to sleep.

PRACTICE: Ending the Day

You can follow along on our website.

Can you end the day with the same intentional quality that you started the day? This can simply be bringing to mind your intentions for the day and asking, with lightness, "How did that go? What went well? What didn't go well, and what can I learn from that?" As we have already covered, a very important part of this can be checking in with a sense of appreciating any moments from the day that you enjoyed, feel went well, or for which you feel grateful. These can be small moments, private moments, or moments with others. Do this with a light curiosity, as if you were talking with a good friend. As you bring these to mind, allow them to really resonate in the mind and body. Then, quite deliberately, let them go.

MOHAMMED: *I take care of my two small children full-time. This means that at the end of the day I normally collapse into bed exhausted. I fall asleep almost as soon as my head hits the pillow—young children can be a great cure for insomnia! When I first tried reviewing my days, it was difficult. The first thing that came to mind was moments where I felt I'd somehow fallen short, been irritable with the kids, not listened to my wife, not got through my to-do list, and so on. If I am honest, it made me feel worse. What helped was the suggestion that I do this like I were talking to a good friend. When I did it like this, I could easily bring to mind moments that brought a smile to my face. The moments my kids chortled as they played, the sense of, yes, relief as I got into the car after dropping them off at nursery, when my wife bathed the kids at night, and I had some time for myself. . . . All I am trying to do—it's simple really, is keep my kids safe and raise them as best I can. When I review my day, I remind myself of this. Mostly I am doing just fine. This helps me sign off and put down the day in a good way. If there were missteps during the day, like I was talking to a friend, I try to be kind and understanding. Sometimes I ask, "Is there anything to be learned?" Through this practice I realized that I used to not want my wife to bathe the kids. I felt it was my job and she was tired after a full day at work, and it wasn't fair to ask her to do this. But I realized this small break in the evening is an important time for her and our kids to connect each day.*

Stopping to review your day and what was good and what went well can enhance your sense of well-being. Of course, you can have bad days. But here too you can start to see that dwelling on the negative tends to make you feel worse and rarely helps with the actual issues. Reviewing things that may have gone wrong in your day with a light, friendly touch and then putting the issues down can help you get to sleep. And often "a bad day" turns out to be a day that had many moments: some will have been difficult—that's why we had a "bad" day—but more than likely if you look carefully enough there will have been moments to appreciate as well.

Mindfulness of Everyday Activities: Taking It Further

As stepping in and out of awareness of everyday activities becomes more natural, you can take this further too. When you spend time with other people, can you really pay attention to what others are saying, verbally and nonverbally? What is your experience in these moments? Do you feel bad, good, safe, scared, connected, disconnected, like you want to be with this person or get away, revitalized or drained?

What about in more charged situations? Can you tune in to how the charge is registering in your body? What is it triggering for you in terms of moods, impulses, and thoughts?

> SAM: When I first tried doing this, I was like, "My life is too crazy busy for this. How am I going to pull this off?" But it turns out, even in the busyness of nursing, and a whole shift can be full-on, there are these little pockets of time where I can check in: bathroom breaks, waiting at the dispensing chemist, in the elevator, at handover team meetings . . .
>
> I figured out in these pockets of time: "All right, I'm gonna take better care of myself during my shift so I don't crash when I get home." And then there was this one crazy day in the ICU with a patient, an Aussie bike courier around my age. He got hit by a garbage truck and was hanging on for dear life. It hit me hard, maybe 'cause we were both in our early 20s, and I bike to work too, usually without a helmet. Plus, he had just landed in the country, knew no one, and I was his only connection as he fought to stay alive. During a bathroom break, out of nowhere I started tearing up. I talked it out with a colleague and we kept checking in throughout the day. Working in the ICU, we're like a tight-knit crew; being affected by the work is just part of the deal. After the shift, my colleague and I grabbed a drink. It helped me shake off the heaviness before heading home. On my way back, I thought, "Hey, I'll phone my parents, just to say hi." They like that, and so do I.

Throughout the day, you can pay attention to everyday activities with a sense of friendly curiosity and interest—beginner's mind. You can raise and broaden your gaze to see more of the world, perhaps noticing things you might not normally see. As you become more familiar with this, you can try it with more charged moments, to see how mind and body register these moments, and also take care of yourself in these moments—as Sam did working on the ICU that day. In fact, I'd like to give the last word to Sam and what went through his mind just before he went to sleep.

> SAM: When I looked back on my day, I realized that even though it was deeply upsetting to see the Australian courier fighting for his life, I knew my nursing had been on

point. I remembered the moments I'd suctioned out the fluid from his throat and placed eye drops in his eyes, taking time to make sure he was as comfortable as possible. He was sedated but distressed, understandably because he was struggling to breathe. I'd talk to him, about nothing and everything. And you know what's crazy? The monitors showed my voice was actually calming his heart rate.

The ICU is this weird mix of intense and quiet, like a spiritual vibe. I knew the deal. I'd find out in the coming days if the courier survived the accident and if so whether he'd have enduring disabilities; but today I had done all I could. I grabbed a drink with my colleague after work and enjoyed the drink, and I messaged her afterward to say, "Thanks for that hug, seriously the best," and she shot back with a smiley hug emoji. I grabbed a take-out on the way home and instead of diving into gaming I ate while chatting with my parents on the phone about nothing in particular. They'd been so pleased to hear from me. They worry about how I am doing, especially with how heavy the ICU can be.

This chapter has invited you to consider the question "How well am I spending my time?" Why is it interesting and important? It makes us pause and reflect on what we say and do. With time, we also become sensitive to the effects of our words and actions, not just on us, but on those around us. For example, a child who breaks something and is asked by a parent what happened might quite automatically expect to get punished and say very quickly, without thinking, "It was already broken when I stepped on it."

Maybe you recognize how easy it is to react like this, even as an adult. Perhaps sometimes words or actions tumble out of you, without your thinking, out of habit, trying to look good, anticipating disapproval, wanting to avoid conflict, and so on.

SOPHIA: *I knocked the mug of tea over and had an automatic reaction of horror and anger, and before I knew it, the words formed writ-large in my head: "You stupid idiot." When I was a girl, there were such high standards in my home. My mother wouldn't tolerate clumsiness, and I would feel so ashamed when I did something wrong. She was always telling us off, or at least it seemed that way. Over time I learned to tell myself off. If I do something "wrong," I react with "Uh-oh, I am going to get into serious trouble. Why am I such a stupid idiot?" It's not just words; there is a real sense of horror, and underneath that, shame.*

Starting your day with a clear intention, trying to stay aware throughout the day, reviewing your day at the end of the day are all ways of answering the question "How well am I spending my time?" You can start to get better at handling your day, so your words and actions don't create problems for you, the people around you, and the wider world. And if they do, you can have the grace and good humor to be honest and straightforward, learning from experience. Over time this leads to a sense of greater confidence in your words and actions and more of a sense of making your own choices.

Waking up and paying attention extends outward to what we do, and don't do, in the wider world. What I mean is waking up can alert us to the well-being of communities and our planet, for example. This theme of widening circles of concern for others and the wider world is one that we'll develop in later chapters.

This chapter has offered you some ways to start and end the day with a sense of intention. But please don't take this as prescriptive. There are many ways of doing this—prayer, running, walking, music, yoga, contemplations, and keeping a diary to name just a few.

Waking Up Every Day, through All Our Days

People usually consider walking on water or on thin air a miracle. But I think the real miracle is to walk on earth. Every day we are engaged in a miracle that we don't even recognize: a blue sky, white clouds, green leaves, the black curious eyes of a child, our own two eyes. All is a miracle.
—THICH NHAT HANH, *The Miracle of Mindfulness*

This quote, from a modest Vietnamese monk who did a huge amount to bring mindfulness into the mainstream, gets to the heart of the matter. I'd add to his list: a spider's web, savoring our food, a coffee mug, being with people we love, the "gaps" in the day, our studies, our work, even doing the laundry. Actually, all the moments of the day.

This chapter has started you off, with waking up and making small changes in how you relate to your day. This includes bringing an attitude of friendly curiosity and appreciation and a sense of "yes" to life. The skill of paying attention is a foundation for all of this. That's what we turn to next.

2

Pay Attention!

What if every day you had an attention budget?
Would you give it all way? Would you spend it
at random?

When you first start practicing mindfulness, it is quite likely you'll have a sense of how distractible, random, scattered, and even chaotic your attention can be. Our minds tend to be filled with whatever is most captivating. Or if it's left to wander, habit takes over and you follow well-worn grooves.

You'd never treat your money the same way, leaving it lying around carelessly, so other people can take it and use it as they wish. And yet that is exactly what we often do with our attention: let other people decide where our attention will be focused. And this costs us. If your attention is constantly drawn to every notification on your phone, for example, you'll likely end up distracted and exhausted. Notifications are designed to capture your attention. If it's social media, you may get sucked into a vortex and absorb whatever your media streams feed you, which will be driven by algorithms designed to first capture and then keep your attention.

Maybe this seems like a radical idea, but you can choose where to place your attention. You can choose to focus on pleasant or unpleasant experience. You can attend to your internal experience or the outside world. You can even choose which sense—seeing, hearing, touching, tasting, bodily sensations—to use.

If some of this seems a long way from where you are, don't worry. In this chapter I'll show how you can train certain attentional skills. You can use these skills to gather your "scattered mind," stabilize, and choose how to use your attention. Attention is a foundational skill for life, one that

> We always start by meeting our mind where it is at and on its own terms.

29

can transform your experience of every day and is essential to planning your future—the next minute, hour, month, year, or stage of life. Take this skill building at your own pace, one step at a time. Remember, this is all about learning mindfulness for life, *for* life.

How Does Attention Help Us in Daily Life?

Our attention is the gateway to all our experience.

What you are paying attention to right now, the words on this page, is your experience in this moment. You are giving these words your complete attention, without being drawn away by distracting input around you just now or intrusive thoughts about what you "should" be doing instead. *Why* are you paying attention to what you're reading? Because you need a break from doing your tax return? Because you've made a commitment to integrating mindfulness into your everyday life? Because you're curious? Attention performs various useful functions in our lives. And many factors can affect it.

The Barefoot Professor: Types of Attention

Amishi Jha, a professor of psychology at the University of Miami, has spent her career studying attention. Her classification of attention as three different types is one useful way of understanding how important this capacity is to our functioning.

Alerting attention: our alarm system. Our mind and body possess an elaborate hardwired alarm system that continually monitors for things that need our attention, mostly things that require a quick, often automatic judgment: pain, threats, unexpected change. It very quickly decides: Is this pleasant, unpleasant, neutral? Do I need to do anything? This alarm system is probably not trainable, but it helps to know that we have a hardwired, automatic alarm system keeping us safe.

Orienting attention: our flashlight. Orienting attention typically follows alerting attention. Once alerted, our attention operates a bit like a flashlight, moving a beam of light onto whatever we're attending to so we can see it in greater detail. When the alarm system goes off, the flashlight reorients: a pang of physical pain, or the car that cut us off on the highway, someone calling our name. But we can also choose to turn the flashlight toward something that we like or want: a message from a friend on our phone, for example (which might take our attention away from reading the words on this page). Finally, we can orient attention outward, to something important that is being said, or inward, to how we feel as we hear it.

Executive attention: juggling. Executive attention is how we work with information, take time to think before acting, resist temptations, plan, reason, choose the information we need, and mentally solve problems. There is so much information to juggle, and this is why Amishi Jha uses the analogy of juggling—we're keeping all these balls in the air, making decisions all the time based on which balls are up and which are dropping down.

Psychology has yielded some important insights about executive attention:

1. *We can only juggle so many balls at a time.* Executive attention takes up cognitive resources, which are limited. Specifically, attention relies on working memory, which has only so much capacity. There is only so much information we can process at any one time.
2. *Our ability to juggle is much worse if we're stressed, our alarm system is activated, we're tired, or intrusive thoughts are pulling on our attention.* A whole range of factors affect our ability to juggle, including how many things are competing for our attention at any one time and our personal history.

Executive attention is something we can become much more familiar with, and I'd argue we can shape it to a significant degree through mindfulness training, although the research on this is still ongoing.

The three types of attention described by the Barefoot Professor probably aren't all directly controllable, but there are ways that you can nonetheless learn to use your attention to help you navigate your life, through meeting routine obligations, responding to crises, and planning to fulfill your dreams.

Attention as Our Protector

Attention serves first as your alarm system, alerting you to imminent danger so you have a chance to take action to protect yourself.

MOHAMMED: *Yesterday I was about to cross the road with my kids, and out of nowhere a car veered dangerously toward me. I grabbed my kids—they hadn't seen the car—and we stepped back very quickly, away from the car's path. Everything else became irrelevant—what we were chatting about, all the surroundings. My attention immediately became focused solely on the car's direction of travel and pulling back my kids and myself onto the sidewalk.*

How often do you forget that your alarm system is a lifesaver? In Mohammed's case, paying attention allowed him to step back and prevent harm to himself and his kids.

But your attention can be protective in other ways. Pain, discomfort in all its forms, fatigue, sleepiness, hunger, thirst, the menstrual cycle's many signals, sexual arousal, thirst, the need to urinate or defecate—they are all calls to pay attention. Attention can also protect you from mental, physical, or emotional overload. During a busy day, or at the end of an overstimulating day, your mind pays attention to the fact that you feel overwhelmed and shuts down or at least shuts out what it can't manage. This can also happen to people like first responders, who work in jobs that expose them to really difficult situations that can be too much to process.

SAM: *After a hard day at work, especially during the pandemic, people throw this question to me: "How are you holding up?" Truth is, more often than not, I'm just kinda numb. It's the only way to deal with some of what I have to see and do.*

In even more extreme circumstances, after a traumatic event, for example, shock is common as the mind shuts down to protect itself. Over a long period of time, overstimulation or chronic stress can lead to mental health conditions such as anxiety, depression, burnout, or even posttraumatic stress. Learning to pay attention to these signs and symptoms enables us to do what we need to look after ourselves.

SOPHIA: *I sat with my mother in the last days of her life. Her mind was closing down as she was drawn into ever more sleep. As her death approached, the sleep became so deep she couldn't be roused. At these times her face and her body seemed to be at ease. I can't be sure, but there seemed to be a very powerful process of changing awareness going on in my mother in front of my eyes. At the same time as I sat with her, all sorts of things were going on for me, including sometimes needing to protect myself when I got upset. I'd go for a walk and there were horses in a field nearby. I'd feed them apples, stroke them, and talk to them about nothing in particular. It was as if there was part of me that knew I needed this to be able to go back into the room to be with my mother.*

Left to its natural wisdom, our mind moves between being present, calls to action, wandering, and, if it feels overwhelmed, protecting itself by taking time out and if necessary, shutting down. This is a natural part of what it means to process all that happens in our days and lives. You can learn to become more familiar with these tendencies of your attention to know when to open and when to protect yourself. The mind, left alone, can do this for itself, but you can come to see it happening, allow it to happen, and maybe even learn when protective awareness does and doesn't serve you.

This is the start of a lifelong journey where you can learn to skillfully deploy your protective awareness.

Attention is a protective gatekeeper. Amid a traumatic event our hard-wired systems take over, our attention automatically alerting to and orienting to what it needs to. But if you start to take control of your attention, you can become a gatekeeper. You can pay attention to who is coming and going but also get better at knowing who is okay to let in and who to keep out—what is good for you and bad for you. This is where mindfulness comes in, particularly the part of mindful attention that is like a flashlight that illuminates what you need to see.

> If attention is the doorway to experience, you need to take care about what you let in.

The Ancient Oak and the Barefoot Professor: Mindfulness as Our Protector

The Ancient Oak: There is an ancient simile of the gatekeeper to a city who is wise, competent, and intelligent, keeping out strangers and letting in people with legitimate business within the city. The gatekeepers maintain the walls, guard the gate, and learn about everyone who comes and goes. They keep the city and all who live there safe.

The Barefoot Professor: Scientists studying attention have explored how the brain controls what we shine the flashlight on and what we filter out. Francis Crick, who also famously worked with James Watson on DNA, proposed that deeper brain structures such as the thalamus act as a relay station, or gatekeeper in your simile, filtering out information. More recently, neuroscientists have turned their attention to brain networks, rather than brain areas, and Michael Halassa, a researcher doing groundbreaking work, showed that networks were connecting different brain areas (prefrontal cortex, specific areas of the thalamus, the basal ganglia—circuits switching on and off), in very sophisticated and subtle ways, both filtering out (gatekeeping!) and highlighting (flashlight) information. This happens when we're awake, but also when we're asleep, when some psychologists believe there is a lot happening, reviewing what has been learned, reorganizing memory, processing what needs processing.

Attention as Our Flashlight

Try watching 24/7 news on a channel that has different views from yours for a few hours and see the effect it has! If you have low-level, chronic pain, try attending to it nonstop. If you're prone to anxiety, try worrying about what you're anxious about without a break. It's exhausting. When you read these suggestions, you probably said, "No way." That's also your protective awareness in action, and, yes, you can trust it. You can start to make choices about what you let in, what you keep out, and how you deal with intruders.

You can take hold of the flashlight and choose where you place your attention (orienting attention). You can also move the flashlight of your attention around, bringing different experiences into focus. You can notice and attend to experiences that are pleasant and unpleasant. And the more you do this, the more confident you'll become in using your attention skillfully (executive attention).

Your Flashlight Has Many Lenses

> Using your flashlight throughout your life reveals that changing lenses changes everything.

"Attention without feeling . . . is only a report," writes the poet Mary Oliver. She suggests that we befriend our attention as an "intentional, unapologetic discriminator."

You can choose different attitudes as lenses for your attention. I've already introduced the attitudes of curiosity and appreciation, but there are other attitudes you can choose as well, such as kindness and care. Most people are not aware of their default attitudinal lens, let alone that they can change their attitude.

> SAM: I hate to own up to this, but my go-to is go with the flow, but in a laissez-faire way. Getting curious about stuff has been a game changer. It sort of lights me up and gives me a bit more oomph.

> SOPHIA: My default lens is to be quite judgmental. I can, like many people, be especially hard on myself—"That's not good enough, Sophia." And, if I am honest, with other people too: "Was she being sarcastic in that text message? Why, she's just mean!"

Try practicing bringing different lenses to your experience, being playful with attitudes of curiosity, appreciation, kindness, and care. You can also change the lenses on your flashlight by swapping in and out each of your senses—bodily sensations, seeing, hearing, tasting, and touching—as lenses.

> LING: If I can't sleep, it's usually because I'm caught up in a vortex of thinking. So, I try, as best I can, to take hold of the flashlight and scan through my body, with a lens that is curious, caring, and tries to stay focused in body sensations.

One of the hardwired properties of attention is its inclination toward difficulties and its tendency to gloss over pleasant experiences.

SOPHIA: *I remember as a kid finding school stressful. There was a lot of pressure from my parents and the school to do well. There were always tests and exams and, in my school, results were posted for everyone to see. I remember always being on the lookout for how to do well academically, and was very alert to mistakes, criticism, and falling short of my teachers' expectations. I'd feel chuffed when I did well, but mostly embarrassed when I didn't do so well. That's probably where a lot of my inner critic comes from. It was a game changer for me to realize that there is a choice—let this inner critic grab attention and overshadow the whole day or refocus on all the parts of the day that have gone well or been enjoyable, allowing that to frame my day.*

Juggling Attention: Multitasking or Task Switching?

Somehow multitasking has become something to aspire to. We see it all around us—students doing homework while listening to music and speaking to someone online. We walk, listening to a podcast, making phone calls, and doing some daydreaming at the same time! At work, our attention might be drawn to messages, the people around us, and for people who work in offices, email is a constant draw on attention. Try this:

EXERCISE: **Task Switching or Multitasking?**

Take the phrase "Attention is the gateway to experience." In your mind, count the number of letters in this phrase and time how long it takes you. How many seconds does this take you?

Now spell the phrase out in your mind, letter by letter ("a, t, t, . . ."). How long does this take you?

Now spell it out in your mind and count at the same time.

There are 33 letters, and it normally takes people 20 seconds or so to count them. Spelling the phrase out usually takes people a few seconds less, but still a fair bit of time. Spelling and counting at the same time usually takes quite a bit longer, certainly not the same amount of time.

What does the multitasking exercise show us? Multitasking is a myth. If the popular myths about multitasking were true, we should be able to do both in the same or less time, but this fundamentally misunderstands attention and memory. Spelling, counting, and reading require mental acrobatics

> We don't multitask. We switch tasks.

(executive control), and doing them at the same time pushes us to our limits. Instead, we switch between reading, naming letters, and counting. That is why it takes longer. We can only do things at the same time when they are so well practiced that we can do them by rote. Everything else needs to be done more intentionally and in turn.

> SOPHIA: *At first I was skeptical about the costs of multitasking. I am a busy person; I often do things at the same time. When I walk my dog, I listen to podcasts and work through problems. When I watch TV, I knit or do the ironing. Someone told me a funny story of how she was watching TV while ironing when the phone rang, and she nearly put the iron to her ear! Thank goodness she caught herself before she burned herself badly.*

We process a huge amount of information automatically and at the same time. But multitasking breaks down if we're doing something new or complex—because it requires a lot of our working memory capacity. Then we need all that working memory for the new task, counting or naming in the exercise above. Also, when we try to do too many things at the same time, we can be prone to mistakes. Finally, asking the mind to continually switch from doing one thing to doing another is tiring and likely to leave us feeling stressed.

> SOPHIA: *When I started to play with these ideas, I realized that, yes, I could do some things that didn't require my full attention, that I knew inside and out, at the same time. Knitting while watching TV was a good example. But I also discovered that giving my full attention to something improved it. If, for example, I went for a walk with my dog Rufus without my phone or a podcast, I enjoyed the walk more, I enjoyed Rufus's company more, saw more, heard more. . . . Sometimes, when I struggle with a problem, and get nowhere, what I have started to do is to put it to the back of my mind (the problem is still there of course), go for a walk, and really let my mind have a rest. Once, I got home, hung my coat back on the hook, and a solution had come to mind. Another time it was not so much a solution as I had a bit more perspective on the problem. I am playing with doing one thing at a time sometimes and seeing what I learn.*

What does Sophia's experience teach us? We can do multiple tasks if we've learned to do them automatically, like knitting or walking. We walk without giving it much attention; but if we're new to walking, as a toddler is, we can't walk and pay attention to something else. I remember the first time my elder daughter walked across a room. I literally held my breath; any distraction would have sent her tumbling. She made it; I was so proud! So, we can maybe listen to a podcast while weeding (if we really know what we're doing with weeding; otherwise, we'll pull up the plants!), or we can watch TV while ironing (if we're very good at ironing). But we couldn't do this if we were new to gardening or ironing.

Training Your Attention

As with any skill, you can train your attention with the right approach and with practice. By intentionally taking control of your attention, you can start to choose where and how to use it. Questions about what to pay attention to, when, and how are complicated; there's no one right answer. If you're in a lot of pain, taking attention away from the painful sensations can be very skillful. But if there is a moment when the body is screaming some important message, like "She likes you!" or "He can't be trusted," it's helpful to listen to these messages.

> Realizing that your attention can be trained gives you the freedom to choose what you attend to, when to attend to it, how to attend to it—and what to do with whatever you discover.

Training Your Attention through Mindfulness Practice

For many people one aspect of modern life is how little they feel in control of their lives. It can be really empowering to know that you can steady and train your attention. Fortunately, you have two avenues to train your attention: through mindfulness practices and in your everyday life.

There are many mindfulness practices that train attention. A good place to start is with the Body Scan, which gathers and grounds your attention in your body.

PRACTICE: **Body Scan**

You can follow the audio on our website.

This mindfulness practice involves intentionally using the flashlight of your attention to scan through your body, tuning in to the sensations in each part of the body in turn. You start by taking a moment to notice where your attention to your body is in this moment. Then take a moment or two to sense your body breathing. Intentionally settle your attention into the body and sense the landscape of sensations within your body in this moment—whether pleasant or unpleasant—and the more muted sensations present in every part of your body. Be mindful of how sensations change moment to moment, ebbing and fading. Explore what it is to steady the awareness within your body—standing or sitting—as your body senses, breathes, listens. Now make a deliberate choice to take hold of the flashlight, move it to the soles of your feet and see what you notice. From here you move up through your body, one part at a time, and notice what you find there.

As you move the flashlight of attention through your body, bring a sense of interest and friendliness to whatever is happening. If you encounter discomfort, even pain, trust your mind, knowing when it is wise to turn away from discomfort and pain and when it is possible to turn toward and gently explore pain. When your mind wanders, which is what minds do, know that a thought is a thought, an image is an image, and return once more to an awareness of the body of the moment, just as it is, without having any expectations.

When to practice the Body Scan: Ideally every day, at least until you have a chance to learn some of its key lessons, maybe in bed just before going to sleep or first thing in the morning.

What you can learn:

- **You become more aware of different aspects of our experience—** bodily sensations; moods; thoughts, images, and thinking (planning, remembering, mind wandering); and impulses.
- **You learn to pay attention in a particular way.** Next time you do the Body Scan practice, ask "How would it be to have a lens of interest and kindness?"
- **You start to develop a greater awareness of your body,** something that is key to using mindfulness skillfully to navigate through your days. This is the what the next chapter will develop further.

Training Your Attention in Everyday Life

Every moment is an opportunity to train your attention. All the lessons learned in mindfulness practices can also be learned and applied in your everyday life. Your mind wanders, you daydream, or worry hijacks you. This can happen when you meditate but also as you go about your day.

As I am writing this, my phone is a constant draw on my attention, with notifications, messages, and so on. I can choose to notice my mind being captured by the notifications and bring it back, with kindness. I can choose to turn the notifications off, turn the phone off altogether, or put it in another room. The draw of my phone is more powerful than the strength of my focus, however, especially if I am tired or stressed. I like the app that my daughter introduced me to, which helps me stay present by setting a timer and blocks my phone for however long I set the timer—usually 30-minute periods at a time. The app plants trees when I have focused enough hours each day, something that I find rewarding and that makes it more likely I'll use it again.

What might help you focus on what's important to you in your day-to-day life?

TROUBLESHOOTING: How to Integrate Mindfulness Practice into Daily Life

Trying to train your attention is like training a puppy. The puppy wants to run off and explore interesting smells; sometimes it ignores your requests and just does as it wants; it takes time to train a puppy. But if you're patient, kind, and consistent over time, the puppy will learn to attend to you, trust you, and respond to your commands. Your attention can also be trained with patience, kindness, consistency, and time.

> There is no free lunch in behavior change: it takes concerted effort, patience, and time.

Mind wandering. When you notice that the mind has wandered, the first thing to do is to meet the mind on its own terms, perhaps saying to yourself, "Minds wander; that is what they do." The next thing is to get curious. Where has it wandered? What is that like? Mind wandering can take so many forms; some are pleasant (reverie), some unpleasant (worry), sometimes useful and sometimes not. We're not talking about reaching some enlightened Zen state; you're simply discovering the nature of your mind. With mindfulness training the invitation is to shift your attention back to where you had intended it to be, with the same kindness and firmness you'd use training a puppy, letting go, as best you can, of any tendencies to rush or judge. You're not doing anything wrong; in fact, becoming aware of mind wandering is part of what you're learning. The puppy isn't wrong to want to play and learn; that's in the nature of puppies. Maybe even congratulate yourself at the moment you notice your mind wandering, be curious about what took it away and where it went, and see if you can be kind to yourself—and playful.

> LING: *You're kidding me, right!? I have to get two teenagers out of bed and to school every morning, I work a full-time job, I have to make sure there is food in the fridge, cook a vaguely nutritious meal in the evening, I haven't had time to clean my house for a month, haven't had a holiday for years, and you want me to do these practices. Really!*

I don't have time. Sometimes you don't have time, and at those instances it is wise to prioritize what needs prioritizing. But it is also good to get curious about the question of what and whom you do and don't make time for in your life. Where does your mental health, your well-being, the well-being of people you love, the wider world fit in? There are always pressing problems that you must attend to, or at least it seems that way. But that's like saying I don't have time to charge my phone battery or fuel my car and then expecting your phone or car to do what you need them too. You need to charge your battery and fuel yourself—it is as foundational for you to live your life as fueling a car. Stress and fatigue make it harder to focus. At these times, give yourself a break. Find a time of day or part of the week when you are most likely to be able to start with a mindfulness practice. Weave the everyday practices in as best you can to your day so they are interesting and useful, not just another thing that adds to your stress.

Feeling like we're doing it wrong or failing. "Doing it wrong" and "failing" are examples of a harsh and judgmental attitude. See if you can be curious and kind in these moments. This is like a clever martial art move. Instead of these harsh judgments striking us, meeting them with kindness deflects their force.

> It is hard to be curious and judgmental at the same time. It is hard to be kind and harsh at the same time.

The Ancient Oak: Learning Without Failing

The conductor and teacher Benjamin Zander describes giving an A to each student in his class who states at the beginning of the course what they want to learn and how they will go about studying. He wants to respect people's intrinsic motivation and remove the fear of assessment that shapes so much student behavior. This is a great metaphor for learning these foundational life skills.

Attention in Real Life, for the Rest of Your Life

> Before now, I've never really valued my attention. But I'm realizing that my attention is the everything through which I experience the world. And now that I can see things more clearly, I'm starting to wonder what I've been mindlessly missing. Perhaps more importantly, what, or who has been missing me?
> —SHANNON HARVEY

Shannon Harvey is an award-winning journalist and filmmaker. She had a wake-up call when she was diagnosed with a serious autoimmune disease with no clear cause or treatment. It threatened her career and her ability to raise her young family. One doctor had even warned it could lead to serious disability, including being unable to walk. Shannon committed to a year of living healthily and made a film about her experiences, *My Year of Living Mindfully*.

One of Shannon's biggest lessons from the year was that her attention was very precious, she barely used it to its potential, and she could learn to train her attention. And that when she did this, everything changed. At first Shannon wasn't sure she could trust the changes, so she recruited a small army of scientists to measure and track any observable changes in her brain and other bodily systems. But over time she realized that her experience was just as important. When she trusted what her own body and mind were telling her directly—that her health status stabilized, she felt calmer, better able to focus on work, more present in her life—it helped her keep her mindfulness practice alive. She came to see her mindfulness practice not as a chore, but as something that maintained these positive changes.

What I noticed as I watched the film of Shannon's year was that while she remained essentially the same person, she was going through a change, meeting her own humanity and the humanity of all the people who were part of her film. There is a scene toward the end when Shannon returns home to Sydney, and her husband and two young children meet her at the airport. In that scene the whole family lights up with a sense of reconnection and love. Integrating mindfulness into our lives can have transformative effects: an increasing awareness of strength alongside vulnerability, potential alongside limitations; the very real challenges of life alongside the capacity for both weakness and resilience; distractedness in the face of a full life, alongside staying connected and engaged, and, above all, love.

Have you ever thought about attention the way Shannon Harvey describes it, as one of our most valuable assets? If your attention was an asset like money, you'd take care of it, keep it safe, and use it well. What would it be like if you treated your attention like your money? Perhaps your life would be enriched— yes, *enriched*. In the rest of this chapter you'll explore how you can develop these skills in attention and focus over months and years. How you can apply them in ever more challenging circumstances. You're going to explore not just how to pay attention, but how to use your attention as an anchor, a doorway, and a protector.

When Your Attention Is Hijacked

Have you ever felt like your attention was hijacked by someone or something outside of yourself? What about those times when you found yourself in another room in your home and couldn't remember why you'd gone there to begin with? Or when you were trying to concentrate on reading an important piece of mail, but your attention kept drifting to what you were going to have for dinner? Maybe you've been in a class or a meeting and didn't hear a word because you were so worried about a loved one's health. We all get stressed, tired, or distracted and have trouble paying attention to things we really need to pay attention to. Feeling as if you have no control over your attention is frustrating, can exhaust you even further, and can leave you feeling tormented by your own thoughts and moods. We don't want to go through life being unable to meet our obligations because we're so scattered. No one wants to miss out on the joy and pleasure of life because we're wandering around in a daze. Even when we've trained our attention through mindfulness practices, we can suffer a temporary loss of the skill—usually just when we need it most. Like when we're trying to listen to the pediatrician describe a serious diagnosis just given to our child and how to treat it. Or when we stay late to pull off a miracle at work despite being burned out. Each stage of life brings new challenges that require us to wield our flashlight adroitly. How can we stabilize and anchor our attention when life seems to be demanding more than we can give?

The Ancient Oak: Anchors

Sailors know that different boats and different conditions need different anchors. What will work for a small boat, in shallow water with a muddy lake bottom in good weather, is different from what is needed for a large boat, at sea, with a rocky seabed and rougher conditions. There are even storm anchors that are used in very heavy storms to keep a boat safe by keeping it head to wind; they do not even attempt to anchor to the ground. Instead, they work by anchoring to the sea itself! This enables the boat to ride the waves and not be broadsided by the storm. It's also more complicated than the type, size, and shape of the physical anchor. Anchors are typically attached to a length of heavy chain, which rests on the sea bottom, preventing the anchor from being tugged directly. The length of rope between the chain and boat is also important; the right length will keep the strain on the anchor manageable and the boat in place.

The point is, you learn that you may need different anchors that you use in different ways depending on the conditions. An anchor can even keep you steady during storms.

Anchoring Your Attention When You Need It

Anchoring attention is a skill that you can use and hone for a lifetime. Here are two simple steps you can take when you need to anchor yourself.

1. Start by noticing the state of your mind and body. Perhaps use a word to describe it.
2. Then very intentionally and deliberately make the decision that you need to anchor yourself. That in this moment pausing and gathering

your attention will help. This means gathering your awareness to a chosen anchor and riding the direct experience of that anchor moment by moment. The anchor is in the foreground. Everything else is still there in a wider awareness—mind states, body states, life circumstances—but the anchor provides a way to stay steady with direct moment-by-moment experience and not get carried away.

Using an Anchor to Match the Situation

The analogy of sailors matching anchors to the conditions holds. This is about experience of what works, which comes through trial and error. When have you needed to gather your attention in the past? What anchors have you found helpful? People most often cite awareness of the feet, hands, breath, ear lobes, and external sounds. Are some anchors more helpful when you feel calm and steady, perhaps your breath in your belly? Are some more helpful when you feel agitated, perhaps sounds around you? Are some more helpful when you're in a stressful situation, perhaps your feet or hands, or even a very stressful situation, perhaps your body moving vigorously? You'll almost certainly learn that you need to adapt how you use the anchor to match the situation. For example, if you're more agitated, changing your posture, so it has a sense of stability and being grounded, may help. Or it may be that you need to slow things down. Perhaps taking a slower, deeper inbreath, counting to five, and then releasing your outbreath through a count of seven. It may be that you need to move, so you're walking or stretching, sometimes slowly or perhaps more vigorously. All of this is in the service of gathering and anchoring your attention. See what you can learn over time about what anchors serve you best at different times.

> SAM: *I've figured out that no matter how crazy my day gets, there are always these moments when I can hit pause and switch things up. It's like checking the weather forecast for my mental state. Earlier today, going up the escalator, I did a quick check-in, and the mental weather report was all about me stressing over the morphine setup ("What if I mess up the dosage? Too little or, God forbid, too much?"). Usually, when I check in, I catch myself zoning out, especially if I'm dead tired or feeling overwhelmed. The trick I've picked up is taking a little weather update. I can switch things around. I can anchor myself. Here's my drill. I pay attention to my whole stance, how I'm standing or sitting, my head, shoulders, arms. And then, boom, I switch things up—I become a ninja. I run a scan through my body, reminding myself I am strong. Now I don't think anyone really notices—but if they do [smiling] they're probably thinking "Who is this ninja nurse?"*

> LING: *When you first asked me to pay attention to my body, honestly, I just felt overwhelmed. So, I decided to look at something in the room, anything really—a vase, or*

a picture, or out a window. Sometimes I listened, just to whatever sounds are around, and that settled me. But over months and years my body has become a sanctuary, not the body that was manhandled, that I was ashamed of. This body, here and now. A sacred, yes sacred, sanctuary.

SOPHIA: *My hands are a useful anchor. I use them for so many important things in my life—art, touch (that's my "love language"), cooking, washing. I simply bring my attention to the sensations in my hands; it's easy, automatic to have a sense of thankfulness for my hands and all they do for me. Throughout the day, when I wash my hands, I take the time to sense the water, soap, and all the movements as they wash each other. In my artwork, I have started to explore "free drawing." When I am unsettled, I sketch whatever comes up as my hand moves across the paper. The movements of my hands and the emerging sketch in front of my eyes gather and anchor my mind at these times.*

Mindfulness for life is a series of steps, each building on the one before. Becoming more familiar with your mind and body is the first step. Then you can start to learn how to anchor yourself at different times and in different circumstances.

Playing with Attention to Enrich Our Lives throughout Life

We often say that children learn through play. But we can all learn through play. Going further with exploring attention involves moving from paying attention to playing with your attention. In a spirit of playfulness, see what works for you, what is interesting, what you enjoy, what gives you a sense of meaning. What happens when you look at something, or just see it in passing? Maybe the alarm system provided by our attention alerts us to danger or something that needs to be fixed or can be ignored. But most of the time what we do immediately if we are not in danger is label what we see; we put it into words. We also make judgments about what we've just labeled: "I don't like that color." "I wish that path wasn't filled with all those weeds."

What if you slowed down and really saw something? A lot of people say it's amazing how fast we make up our minds about what we see. It's great that we can quickly label everything—chair, table, friend, tree. But this immediacy can miss the richness of our senses. By slowing everything down, and taking control of your attention, you can open to colors, shapes, and brightness and really see them. Babies learn to do this in the first few years of life. When you choose to see like this, you come closer to the way babies are learning to see the world, for the first time, in all its wonder. And you can start to see the point at which your perception trips into labeling everything. Try this:

PRACTICE: Seeing

The Mindfulness for Life website provides guidance.

This is a practice in seeing afresh. It involves choosing something to look at, out-side or inside. It doesn't matter too much what it is—anything will do—but it helps to choose a focal point and then steady your attention on that focal point. What you're doing here is trying to see the object in terms of colors, shape, shade, patterns, and movement. What exactly is the color as you see it? Is the color steady, or does it change and morph? What people invariably discover is that our mind rushes ahead to summarize the experience—"This is x or y" or "I know what this is." It is practic-ing seeing with childlike curiosity—being open to whatever the flashlight of attention shines its light on. And you can extend this practice by broadening the flashlight into a floodlight, so the whole field of what you are seeing becomes the object of attention. (Adapted from Christina Feldman and Willem Kuyken, *Mindfulness: Ancient Wisdom Meets Modern Psychology* (Guilford Press, 2019, p. 35)

Psychologists discovered decades ago that seeing is not actually like a camera; it is much more like a production suite: we touch images up, fill them in, add in detail. But more than this we create stories . . . it is a creative process! You don't really see things as they are; you see things based on your experience and how you are in this moment. This means that if you feel really hot or cold, are very hungry or thirsty, have traveled across time zones and feel disoriented, or have some condition like an ear infection that affects your sense of balance, your sensory experience is going to be very attuned to that, to the point that it can dominate your awareness. (If you desperately need to pee, can you really pay attention to anything else?)

Once you've gathered your scattered mind and learned to anchor your attention, you have a chance to play with your attention, with friendliness and curiosity. You can choose to open to new vistas. When you do this, new doorways open.

SOPHIA: *I was walking along the Thames with my partner, who is an art collector; we'd just been to an art exhibition. At one point he stopped, and we looked at the river—I guess in the same way we'd looked at some of the paintings. It was late winter/ early spring, and it had rained a lot, so the river was running full and fast. There were so many colors and shades in the river—browns, greens, even yellows. The water's surface was moving, and in many ways, with small and large eddies, and toward the bank there were back eddies. The winter sun, low in the sky, was casting shadows on the water, that you had to do a second take to see. In short, there was so much to see, which until he stopped I had barely noticed. Right there, next to the tow path, it was like looking at an impressionist painting, but it had come to fully animated life; it was beautiful, interesting, textured, and it changed moment by moment. I slipped my hand*

into his and we walked hand in hand, with a real sense of intimacy not only with the
world around us, but with each other too. He approached the whole walk with a curios-
ity that was catching. I had done that walk many times, but he brought an energy and
vividness to moments that I would have let slide by unnoticed.

Sophia is describing this developing capacity to see the world afresh, seeing more, in greater detail, as though our attention is like a telescope becoming
ever more powerful. Awareness is penetrating, but also open. It can be quite
bodily, a sense of being at one or "moved," perhaps to tears of joy, or deep
calm, or a call to action. By recognizing and savoring these moments you can
broaden and build a sense of appreciation, happiness, and gratitude. Attention is a form of generosity. For example, you appreciate a moment of connection with someone you care about, and that develops the relationship and your
sense of connection with that person. Think about a time you felt someone
was really giving you their undivided, 100% attention; they wanted to see you,
understand you. What was that like? By choosing to pay attention, this is what
you are doing, for yourself and for others too.

Playing with our attention can over time help us see things more clearly
and with more detail. Eating is a good example; slowing down and paying
attention to eating means you can really taste, smell, and savor your food.

MOHAMMED: *My kids are becoming fussy eaters, and last week I was trying to decide*
on what to cook for dinner and one kid said, "No, I hate that," and to my next sug-
gestion the other said, "No, I don't like that." That went on to pretty well everything I
suggested. So, I suggested we play a game over the weekend, a tasting game. They were
reluctant, but agreed as long as I didn't feed them broccoli or cabbage. So, blindfolded
they had to guess what everything was, and they got a point if they got it right, and they
had to give a thumbs up, down, or sideways on whether they liked it. They got a sip
of water between samples. I started with some very plain savory food, couscous, sweet
corn, then something a bit more flavored, home-made shakshuka, with a sauce that
sneakily includes other vegetables (no broccoli or cabbage, I promise), then some sweet
food (chopped dates), homemade sweet potato chips, several samples of chocolate, and
finally two flavors of ice cream. They didn't dislike anything, and they weren't able to
guess what food they were getting most of the time, instead having to use words like
mushy (sweet corn), crunchy (my homemade chips), cold and yummy (ice cream, obvi-
ously) and so on.

Mohammed's food tasting with his kids enabled them in a fun way to get
past their immediate judgment, "I hate vegetables," to tasting, smelling, and
otherwise sensing food. Attention, imbued with curiosity, is something they

already had in other areas of their life—the walk to school, looking for bugs in their back garden—and they were now applying it to eating.

All our senses work in more or less the same way. The sense organ (eye, ear, nerve endings in the body, tongue) picks up the raw data and turns it into something the brain and body can work with. You then turn it into something that makes sense and integrate it with whatever else is going on and your previous experience. While our senses work in broadly the same way, we rely on some more than others. We use seeing a great deal to make sense of the world, and this is reflected in the complexity of the eye, the visual cortex and the neural networks involved in vision. We never just look at one thing; we are always differentiating what is in the foreground, what is in the background, how far away something is, if it's moving and if so in what direction, where we are in relation to what we're looking at. Infants see their world with much of this complexity well before they can use language. If we see people on a hill in the distance, we also know we can be seen from that hill. Compare this to touch and imagine or shut your eyes and ears and pick up and touch an object. Touch is about temperature, contours, size, and texture, but it does not really include perspective, at least not in the same way. Each sense has a different function. Just as pressure of water in the ocean turns sediment to limestone, your attention transforms what's happening in your senses into your lived experience—the empowering message is that you can play a role in this process.

Paying Attention for Life

Attention can be an alarm system, a protector, a flashlight, an anchor, and a way of opening new doorways. Learning skills in attention can seem like a big ask. It is, but we know from both ancient wisdom and modern psychology that we can train our attention. And when you do, you see things afresh, have a greater sense of control, and are able to align your attention with what is important both in your life and in the wider world.

3

Coming Home to Our Bodies

Mr. Duffy lived a short distance from his body.
—JAMES JOYCE

How much of the day would you say you have a sense of your body? Do you feel your body is somewhere "you can come home to"? Or do you, like Mr. Duffy in James Joyce's *The Dubliners*, live some distance away?

MOHAMMED: *At school, sports were my life. My dream was always to be a professional athlete. As I went through school, each season was better than the one before. I really felt like I was inching closer to my dream. I love sports; for years it was my life. When I got the letter offering me a full college sports scholarship, it was as if all my dreams had come true. But in my junior year at college my dreams came crashing down. I had a career-ending spinal injury. As if that wasn't hard enough, I had to learn to live with the back pain from the injury. My body had let me down. My body went from being something I knew and trusted to being something that gave me constant pain.*

When you first asked me to do a Body Scan, I thought, "It's ridiculous to ask me to feel my pain. Why would I do that? You're kidding, right?" I really didn't want to do it. I had learned to shut off my body, try to get away from the pain. In those first few Body Scans, the pain in my back tugged on my attention. I remember having the thought, "I'd rather be getting on with all the things that need doing." I had this rising sense of impatience and uptightness.

LING: *I hated it, every moment of it. I think I hate my body. . . .*

SAM: *My mom always called me "Skinny Sam" as a boy; it was affectionate—I was naturally very slight. Fast forward to puberty, and I hit a phase where I was super self-conscious and not exactly bursting with confidence. It seemed like every boy in my year worked out in the gym, played sports, or was just naturally athletic; or maybe it just*

48

seemed that way. I was 100% sure boys that looked like me were just not fit. My room didn't have a mirror, and I avoided looking in mirrors, especially when I didn't have any clothes on. When I first did a Body Scan in a mindfulness class, my brain had this knee-jerk reaction: "Really! I have to pay attention to my body, Skinny Sam? Nobody else does, so why should I?"

SOPHIA: *With each decade, my 30s, 40s, 50s, I found it hard to accept the changes in my body: postkids stretch marks and a belly that was never quite the same, aches and pains in my Achilles and shoulder. Menopause was hell, way worse than I expected. Why the hell didn't someone warn me? The Body Scan at first was just a torrent of these thoughts, with occasional mini breaks as I tried to settle my attention, tried, mostly unsuccessfully, to be kind and patient.*

Like Mr. Duffy, many of us don't fully inhabit our bodies. Why should we? Like Mohammed, Ling, Sam, and Sophia, we don't always like what we find there. I've raised two daughters and discovered that young women's bodies are idealized and objectified (and there's plenty of evidence that the same is true for young men these days). There is a painful gap between how they feel their bodies should be and how they experience them. There are lots of norms telling us that athletic prowess, beauty, youth, and perfect health are what make us okay. So we create stories about how our bodies should be, often with a sense that we're falling short and our bodies have let us down. They are not as athletic, thin, youthful, or sexy as they should be. We're all a bit scared of getting sick and getting old—or maybe even terrified.

But our bodies do so much for us. Think about this: In an average lifespan, you'll take about 500 million breaths, extracting life-giving oxygen from the air, spreading it through an incredibly complex system of blood vessels to every one of the more than 25 trillion cells in your body. You don't have to remember to breathe; it's managed deep in our brainstem by networks of neural activity working together to control our breathing rhythm. This tells our abdominal muscles and diaphragm to drive the inbreath and the outbreath. These muscles are powerful because our large brains need lots of oxygenated blood. I bet you didn't know this: you take a large breath—a sigh—every five breaths or so as the body demands a particularly large amount of oxygen.

Our breathing is tied in to pretty much everything in our body, our level of activation, pupil dilation, and all our senses. Our breathing is also closely tied to all our emotions. This has two major implications. Our breath tells us how we're doing. And intentionally changing our breathing is part of changing our state of mind and body.

Our bodies are a deep source of rich information, a readout of our health and well-being and much, much more. Our hearts will beat about 3 billion times, pumping blood filled with essential nutrients through our arteries and veins. Our complex immune systems will relentlessly find and neutralize pathogens.

Thanks to your brain, you have an extraordinary capacity for learning. A fetus's brain grows at an astonishing rate of about 250,000 nerve cells per minute through the course of pregnancy. Babies, toddlers, and children accumulate an incredible amount of new information, as well as the ability to use that information to balance, walk, use language, form relationships, and so on. Our minds will process an unfathomable amount of input throughout our lives, supported by the 3-pound organ that is the human brain. Our adult brain is made up of billions of neurons, sending and receiving information through our nervous systems, some at the same speed as a Formula 1 car (about 360 km per hour), across an estimated 100 trillion or so interconnections.

Stop and really think about your body and mind doing all of this.

So, why would you want to come home to your body? Because if you can learn to pay attention to your body, really tune in, and become intimate with it, there is so much you can learn. Your body can become your teacher, your sanctuary, your home, and your friend.

In this chapter you're invited to explore how you relate to your body, how you can learn to embrace all it offers, and how coming home to your body can help you throughout your life.

Your Body Is an Anchor, a Teacher, and a Guide

Paying attention, explored in the last chapter, helps us see that we can always gather our minds, however busy our lives are, in our breath and body. When you start to pay attention to your body, one of the first things you notice, in fact, is that apart from moments of strong distress (pain or illness) or great pleasure (sensual pleasure or delicious food), you're normally not very aware of your body.

Try this mindfulness practice.

PRACTICE:	Noting the Body's Climate

You can follow along on our website.

Pause and turn the flashlight of your attention to your body. How is your body right now? Maybe scan your body from your feet, up through your legs, pelvis, torso, hands, arms, shoulders, neck, and head. Note any sensations in the body, whether they are pleasant, unpleasant, or neutral. No need to try to change anything; simply note any sensations in your body. Try to allow any sensations to be exactly as they are. Any sensations of discomfort or any pleasant sensations, or any parts of your

> body that seem to have nothing much going on? Is there any overall sense, in this moment, of calm or agitation, safety, or feeling anxious, able to stay with this moment or impatience, wanting to rush on?

Deliberately turning the flashlight of attention on your body in this interested and nonjudgmental way is quite new for many people. What did you find? You might have been surprised to find out what you can learn in this single moment. Mindfulness of the body is always a present-moment practice. You don't experience yesterday's sneeze or tomorrow's tiredness. You only have whatever you're experiencing in your body right now. If you don't open the body door, you may miss it. The climate of your body wafts away like the breeze that brushes your face for a second and then moves on. With it goes the scent of a flower that just bloomed (or the garbage that needs to be emptied), the smell of rain in the air, or the sudden drop in temperature that tells you it's time to go indoors.

If you pay attention, you can learn how your body is giving you an update on the state of your health and well-being.

The Barefoot Professor: Lighting Up Our Bodies with Awareness

Lauri Nummenmaa, director of the Human Emotion Systems laboratory at Finland's University of Turku, asked hundreds of people what was happening in their bodies when they experienced different states and emotions—anger, fear, disgust, love, depression. He used their responses to draw color maps showing where in the body and how intensely these different emotions are experienced. We can learn so much from these body maps. The face, shoulders, torso, and belly are key to many emotions, lit up brightly in states of arousal (fear, love) and pretty dark in states such as depression. The hands and pelvis also feature, but with more subtlety. His research group has also gone on to look at how these states register in the brain, using brain-scanning technology, and in the body, using measures such as heart rate, skin temperature, and responsiveness. Many emotions share a similar brain and bodily template along axes of arousal (low to high arousal) and valence (positive to negative). This fascinating work invites an exploration of how you experience these states and emotions in your body.

Are You Thinking or Experiencing as You Move through the World?

We all use different modes of mind to make sense of what happens in our daily lives from moment to moment. The mode of mind you probably know best is *thinking about* what's happening and using words to describe it. The thinking mode is how we plan, educate ourselves, get a job, learn from our mistakes, and so on. It's how we create the story of our lives. It's what enabled Sam to study to become a nurse and Sophia to teach her students. At its best, thinking is where we can be creative and plan. We can create and re-create the world in our imagination. With the thinking mode we've figured out how to send humans into space, create complex digital technologies, form historical narratives, and concoct philosophies, and will address the challenges of pandemics, human migration, and climate change.

While a great help, thinking can also be a problem.

The writer Mark Twain joked, "I have been through some terrible things in my life, some of which actually happened." So many issues in our lives can easily be made worse if we overthink them. When we can't sleep and we start thinking "I'm so frustrated . . . I need to sleep . . . why can't I sleep? . . . oh no, tomorrow I am going to be so tired," we simply wind ourselves up and make it more difficult to sleep. When somebody does something we don't understand, we ask ourselves, "What did they mean by that?" We turn it over in our mind, but we'll never be able to read their mind, so it's all just guesswork.

These sorts of problems often need a different response, one that doesn't involve thinking. Take falling asleep; it involves letting go. With misunderstandings, the only way to find out why someone did something is to ask, and even then, we can't be sure they'll tell us—they may not even know themselves or want to tell us!

Sometimes we have to accept not knowing and uncertainty. Sometimes, instead of thinking, we need careful listening and empathy. Sometimes, instead of thinking, we need to let something go because it's not that important. Sometimes a rapid response is needed, with little time to think. Or the best response is an intuitive one, not a rational one.

There is another mode of being in which we experience the world more directly, in the present moment, with all its detail and richness, be that our inner world of sensations, moods, impulses, or thoughts or our outer world. In this mode, experiences unfold moment to moment without being elaborated by thinking about them or turning them into words or ideas. A sensation is simply a sensation, a mood a mood, an impulse an impulse, a thought a thought. It's much more bodily; we're much more in touch with our senses and what's happening in our bodies, moment by moment. I'll call this the *experiencing* mode. This mode is always available to us. We can gather our minds, stabilize our attention, and choose to step into experiencing at any time.

Why would we do this? Because it allows us to savor many positives in life, like the sun on our face, the way music makes us feel, the touch of a loved one, or the taste of food. It can also powerfully connect us to negative emotions, sensations, and experiences, of physical pain or emotions like anger and fear.

We develop a real intimacy with our bodies in experiencing mode. Intimacy is a word sometimes reserved for lovers, or if not for lovers, relationships that have depth. But it can be just the right word for our relationship with our body. With a new friend or lover there is a process of getting to know them, learning over time what they like and don't like, their strengths and vulnerabilities, what has made them who they are today. It's the same with our bodies. This learning, like any learning, takes trial and error and time.

Because the experiencing mode evolved to support our survival, it is very good at making sense of social situations, providing us with a sense of the dynamics of a group, for example. It can give us what is sometimes called a "gut sense," or intuition about a situation.

> ### The Barefoot Professor: Experiencing Mode of Mind
>
> Experiencing as a way of understanding is something we share with other species, and none of us would have survived without it. Throughout our evolutionary history we—and other species—had to continually register and respond to cues about the state of our internal and external world to adapt and survive for another day . . . and another generation. We and other social animals—a herd of gazelles in the African savannah, a pack of wolves in Siberia, a pod of dolphins in the ocean, or an unkindness of ravens in the English countryside—are always learning what to do to stay safe and connected with others. It's a deep form of learning that enables us to respond, intuitively, without thinking and to ensure that as individuals, families, and herds or tribes we remain safe, watered, fed, and so on.

Is experiencing mode always appropriate? Always preferable to thinking mode? Obviously not. We need to be able to plan and analyze, and for that we need to think. We also may not always want to immerse ourselves in experiencing—such as in very challenging situations, when it might be overwhelming to be in touch with our bodies and minds. People with histories of mental health problems and/or trauma may have understandably learned to avoid this mode of mind because it brings up strong negative memories and emotions.

Mindfulness for life is about developing a real familiarity with the landscape of your thinking and experiencing mind and body. You can see that these modes of mind are ways of knowing that serve you in different ways, at different times, and in different situations. When is it easy to think about or directly experience the world, and when is it difficult? When is it wiser to use your experiential model, and when your thinking mode? Can you move seamlessly between them, or even hold both?

Keeping Our Body in Mind
and Our Mind in Our Body

Our minds and bodies are completely interconnected. Everything that happens in our body is in some way registered in our mind, and all our thoughts have an imprint on our bodily systems. We need to take advantage of both thinking mode and experiencing mode throughout life. Mindfulness can keep us from getting stuck in thinking mode, as we modern humans are likely to do, but also can help us stay informed by our experiences so that we gain a fuller understanding of what's going on with us and our world. We may toggle back and forth seamlessly between experiencing and thinking, so that we can check in with our moment-to-moment experience and also shift into thinking mode whenever needed. It's helpful to conceptualize these two moods as separate, but in our daily lives keeping our body in mind and our mind in our body go on together, entwined, like two strains of music in a symphony.

> MOHAMMED: *I remember spending time with coaches and psychologists, who would give me feedback on my training and performance. They helped me when I was out with various injuries. I learned very early on that sports were as much mental as physical. They used to talk about tiny marginal gains in fitness, strength, and performance in competitions. But there were also massive gains to be made in how I approached training, how I dealt with pressure, setbacks, peers. When I was doing well, I was more relaxed, and I noticed that when I was more relaxed this helped recovery and set me up for the next training sessions. If I had thoughts pop into my head like "I'm not good enough; this is going to be a terrible session," it affected my performance—somehow my body felt less responsive, slower.*

The body is incredibly sensitive both to what's happening in our minds and in the wider world. It picks up things before we're even aware of them. Professor Lisa Feldman-Barrett has provided compelling evidence for what she calls "affective realism." Stress, tiredness, and negative emotions can lead to our losing perspective. In other words, our emotional state powerfully shapes what we think. If we're feeling tired, maybe after a sleepless night, it's harder to concentrate, easier to make mistakes, and we're more prone to feeling emotional. The good news is that when we start to recognize this, we can do something about it.

> MOHAMMED: *If I was about to compete, I used strategies to recognize and let go of self-sabotaging thoughts. Over time they became less frequent. I developed routines that got me into a frame of mind—and body—to compete. These were stretches and warm-up*

routines, but I also learned to really tune in to my body as I was doing them so I could adjust what was needed. My body, as the expression goes, really was my temple.

Chronic Stress: A Mental and Physical State

Chronic stress is an extreme example of this feedback loop. There is now a lot of evidence that chronic stress is much more than a mental state; it is made up of mental and bodily states. The sense of threat and feeling overwhelmed floods the body with neurotransmitters and hormones that create states of arousal—a readiness for action. Our bodies are hardwired to react to challenges, but when the stress passes it is also hardwired to return to its resting state. Chronic stress keeps it in this state of hyperarousal, which is fine short-term, but long-term starts to cause damage because systems in our bodies become *inflamed*. The word *inflamed* calls up images of fire, soreness, pain, and swelling, and inflammation is associated with many long-term health conditions. We're starting to see the short- and long-term damage this can do in terms of health behaviors, such as overeating, and health outcomes—hypertension, diabetes, for example. The good news is that mindfulness training has been shown to help with these conditions in terms of our mental health but also in some early research in terms of some physical health outcomes, like hypertension. One possible way it does this is to interrupt this cycle of inflaming our stress response long-term, teaching us to spot when this is happening and to do something different.

Avoiding chronic stress is only one of many reasons to train ourselves to learn from our bodies and to become comfortable working with body–mind feedback loops.

Learning to Come Home to Your Body

Awareness of your body, learning to recognize and switch between thinking and experiencing, is something you can do in every area of life. Here's a great start:

Listening to Music

Listening to music, something many of us do (and enjoy) in our daily lives, is a good way to feel the difference between experiencing and thinking. Read through the instructions and then have a go.

PRACTICE: **Listening to Music in Two Ways**

You can follow along on our website.

Choose a song or piece of music you like, that is meaningful to you, that makes you feel something. Settle yourself into a comfortable position.

Start the music, and as you listen, *think about the music*. What thoughts come up? Why is it meaningful to you? Is it the way you remember it—better, worse, the same? Who wrote the music? Who is performing it? When was it written? If you had to describe it to someone in words, how would you do that? After a while, perhaps a minute or longer if you prefer, pause the music. What did you notice? What happened for you?

Restart the music and this time *allow the sounds to come in through your ears. Can you sense the sounds in your mind and body?* Let the sounds run through you and feel any feelings that come up, simply experiencing the music and any sensations as they are. When you notice yourself thinking or judging what's happening, recognize that and let it go, come back to the simple experience, moment by moment, of the music.

What did you notice in the first part, when you were thinking about the music? What about the second part, when you were experiencing the music? What was different about being in the two modes?

People often say that when they allow themselves to simply experience the music it touches them; that it resonates emotionally. Thinking about the music and describing it in words can help us see things about the music, but it also tends to turn off the sense of connecting with it emotionally. People who are musicians have told me they switch between both modes, each informing and enhancing the other—for example, feeling sad in one part and then happier in another—and that the music has switched from a minor to a major key. Others have commented that you can relate to music in ways that transform the experience (for example, sitting in a classical concert hall, a religious setting, dancing wildly in front of the stage at a concert, relaxing comfortably in your living room).

You can try the same experiment with shifting between experiencing and thinking in how you relate to art, the natural world, and pretty well every aspect of your life. Try it for yourself as you move through your day.

Mindfulness Practices for Inhabiting Your Body

Many mindfulness practices train us to keep our body in mind. The three main body-focused mindfulness practices are the Body Scan, Mindful Movement, and Mindful Walking, all of which essentially do the same thing: help you get used to more fully inhabiting your body. I introduced the Body Scan in Chapter 2 because it starts you off doing this at rest. Here you'll proceed to moving.

The Body Scan. The Body Scan is a practice you can return to again and again, as you learn to really inhabit and stay with whatever you discover in your body. It can be practiced for a few minutes as a way of coming into your body or for longer—10–30 minutes or more.

Mindful Movement. This practice builds on the Body Scan, taking you through a series of simple movements in which you inhabit your body. Pleasant and unpleasant sensations will come and go, and you can see how you relate to these. Is it possible to stay with sensations, without holding on to them or pushing them away, with a spirit of interest and care? The invitation is very simple. Intentionally, slowly move through these postures. Practice again and again, bringing your attention to your body. You can find full instructions and videos on our Mindfulness for Life website.

Mindful Walking. Most of us walk from place to place without giving it much thought. This practice asks you to walk deliberately and with awareness.

PRACTICE: Mindful Walking

You can follow along on our website.

Is there a stretch of corridor, pavement, or footpath that you walk each day? Make this your (secret!) walking path. Each day, when you walk this stretch, make this shift in how you approach it: Pay attention to the soles of your feet and/or the movement of your feet and legs. Instead of looking around or daydreaming or planning whatever is coming up in your day, rest your awareness in your body as it walks. That's all. When the mind wanders, gently escort it back. Use the sensations in your feet and legs as an anchor connecting you to the present moment.

This is—obviously!—a very movable practice. You can do it anytime and anywhere you're walking. It can be very grounding to anchor yourself in the soles of your feet, your legs, your whole body, walking. To give thinking a rest.

What Can You Learn from Body-Focused Practices?

These body practices are extraordinary teachers. They very likely will bring up your habits and all the ways that you normally relate to not just your body but also your life.

MOHAMMED: *I discovered strength and vitality in my body that I hadn't really noticed before. I am still fit, relatively young, strong; I work out in the gym in my basement most days. This helped me enjoy these gym sessions more. Rather than being something I did out of habit, or had to do, it became something I looked forward to and enjoyed, a chance to enjoy being in my body as I worked out and not think about all the have-to-dos in my life.*

LING: *My body was screaming out to tell me all sorts of things about my state of mind. It was almost like my body was saying "Why have you been ignoring me? I need some looking after." It was telling me, "Yes, you have a very active mind; it makes you light up—iridescent is the word I would use. But I am a more reliable indicator of where you're at, when you're scared and when you're feeling safe, connected, or disconnected, and so on. Let's be friends."*

Most people discover that how they approach this practice is how they approach their lives. People who tend to strive bring striving to the practices: "I need to get this right." People who tend to be self-doubting might put it off or abandon it after concluding, "I don't think I can do this." You can explore these tendencies in the practices. Just notice these thoughts: "Ah, there you are, striving" or "I see you doubt, I am calling you out."

When you move, you also meet boundaries and limits. How do you tend to react to boundaries and limits—try too hard, don't try hard enough, think it's too easy, too hard, a competition with yourself or others? It's likely you'll approach the movement practice the same way. You can use all that you learn in these practices to inform how you take care of yourself in your life.

MOHAMMED: *I approached these practices the way I'd approached my fitness plan as an athlete, a project to get right and to improve myself. When I first saw that I was doing this, I could step back and practice just being in my body without trying to change anything. After all, I am not an athlete anymore and there is nothing I have to achieve here. My back injury had already been an exercise in accepting new limitations; so now I tried kindness and care instead of striving and being the best I can be. It was sort of eye opening; I could see the many parts of my body that don't function so well, with kindness and friendliness. It also brought home to me that actually there is a lot right with my body.*

One of the most important early lessons from these practices is how you could take better care of your body. Paying attention in this way helps you know when your mind and body need something. As you become more tuned in, you can start to ask questions like "What do I need right now?" and "What keeps me healthy?" and "How can I make this self-care a part of my life?"

SAM: *I got into the habit of doing a Body Scan at the end of the day and would always fall asleep. Turns out, I was way more exhausted than I realized. Instead of beating myself up—"I have to do this Body Scan"—I cut myself some slack and went to bed earlier—I needed the sleep and rest big time. I had an inkling that I had to look at my sleep habits and get more and better sleep. I researched a good sleep app, I found one with lots of evidence, and downloaded it. It started by looking at my sleep and made suggestions about a more regular bedtime and not using my bedroom for gaming or scrolling through social media. Over weeks and months, I changed some of my habits and routines. Changing my habits and routines, especially for someone as set in their ways as me, wasn't a walk in the park. But hey—it worked. Why? 'Cause each day, I noticed I was feeling more upbeat, brighter. That made sticking to the changes and turning them into new habits a whole lot easier.*

The Barefoot Professor: What Our Bodies and Minds Need

Psychologists know quite a lot about what supports our well-being, and it's not rocket science. Well-being is maintained by:

- Adequate sleep
- A healthy diet
- Exercise
- Positive social connections
- Doing things that give us a sense of accomplishment and that we enjoy.

In the same way we "practice" a sport or a musical instrument to get better at it, we can practice doing what supports our well-being.

The Breathing Space

Early in this chapter I emphasized the importance of the breath to our bodies and minds. If you've done any mindfulness training, you likely learned (or at least heard of) the Breathing Space. The Breathing Space is a take-anywhere mindfulness practice that taps the power of the breath. It can help us immediately come home to our bodies by taking a pause and using that pause, during which you fully inhabit the body, to reset. It opens up doorways that give a sense of choice and freedom in any moment. For example, like the other body-focused mindfulness practices, the Breathing Space can help you recognize the need for self-care.

> The Breathing Space is the one new skill that many people really build into their lives once they learn it, because its power to make a real difference to their lives is immediately evident.

Maybe you just need to stretch, or you need to get out of the office and take a walk outside the building.

PRACTICE: The Breathing Space

You can follow along on our website.

Step 1. Becoming Aware

Become more aware of how things are in this moment by deliberately adopting an upright and dignified posture, whether sitting or standing, and, if possible, closing your eyes. Then bring your attention to whatever you are experiencing right now, asking:

- What body sensations are here right now?
- What moods and feelings are here?
- What thoughts are going through my mind? Is there any imagery around?
- Are there any impulses or calls to action right now?

Step 2. Gathering

Then redirect your attention to focus on physical sensations associated with breathing. Bring the mind to settle on the breath, wherever you feel it most vividly. Tune in to these sensations for the full duration of the inbreath and the full duration of the outbreath.

Step 3. Expanding

Then expand your attention around the breath, so that it includes a sense of the body as a whole, your posture, facial expression, your torso, the whole of your body.
    As best you can, bring this wider awareness to the next moments of your day.

Adapted from J. Teasdale, M. Williams, M., and Z. Segal, *The Mindful Way Workbook: An 8-Week Program to Free Yourself from Depression and Emotional Distress* (The Guilford Press. 2014), p. 183.

What Can You Learn from the Breathing Space?

The Breathing Space enables you to gather your mind, whatever state your mind is in—scattered, jangled, agitated, sleepy, alert, upset, elated, calm, downhearted. You become better and better at recognizing and labeling your experiences, from physical sensations, to moods, impulses, and thoughts. You learn that you can always "anchor" your attention and which anchors work best at which times. Sometimes the best anchor is the feet, sometimes the hands, sometimes the breath. You learn to intentionally shift out of autopilot and to move between thinking and experiencing modes of mind or to have a sense of both modes in broader awareness. Finally, the Breathing Space is always available as a way to recognize, allow, anchor yourself, and step back from what is happening. We'll return to it over and over.

The Barefoot Professor: Using the Breathing Space to Measure Your Arousal

In her classic book *How Emotions Are Made*, Lisa Feldman Barrett explains that we can understand how we are doing in any given moment along two dimensions, valence (pleasant or unpleasant) and arousal (awake, sleepy, or something in between). For example:

> High arousal, pleasant—elated, thrilled
> High arousal, unpleasant—angry, anxious
> Low arousal, pleasant—at ease, calm
> Low arousal, unpleasant—fatigued, depressed

Assessing valence and arousal can be helpful as we start to tune in to Step 1 of the Breathing Space. Then, in Step 2 you can get an index of your arousal by noticing whether your breath is shallow or deep, irregular, or steady. While the breath is controlled deep in the nervous system, you can also bring it under conscious control, at least to a degree. . . .

TROUBLESHOOTING: Sticking with Inhabiting Your Body So It Becomes Integrated into Your Daily Life

The preceding practices are not difficult to do in and of themselves, but sometimes you'll encounter stumbling blocks. Because these practices are so key to experiencing through your body—and therefore so powerfully useful in daily living, throughout life—it's worth sticking with building these skills,

Discomfort and pain. What stops many people from learning the skills of coming home to their body is that it can highlight unpleasant sensations or even intensify them. If this happens, keep in mind that anchoring your attention means you won't get carried away by these sensations and thoughts. You can bring kindness and care and ask, "What do I need in this moment?" Chapter 9 offers resources you can use to get around this stumbling block and keep coming home to your body.

Does paying attention to your body feel "stupid and self-indulgent"? We're used to how things are. We prefer being lost in thought, reminiscing about the past and fantasizing about and planning the future. If our bodies are something we're not comfortable with or don't like—too thin, too fat, too short, too tall, don't work as well as they used to—it may feel counterintuitive to pay attention to them.

> Most of us have bought into the idea that unless it demands our attention, what's happening in our body is a sideshow at best.

To get around this obstacle, learn to listen carefully to what your body is saying, in the same way you'd listen to a good friend. Messages like "This sensation feels good; this bit is tingling; this hurts; you're not ready to tune in to this or do this stretch, back off; this is interesting, pay attention carefully" can be an invitation to move into something and explore it more fully. What you'd always labeled as "my painful knee" turns out to be a whole range of different sensations. Trust yourself. If your mind is saying "Take care, back off," listen to it—you're bringing a protective awareness to what is happening. You can always come back to something later or break it into bite-sized pieces.

If you feel uncomfortable with your body, one way of disarming the discomfort is through humor.

SAM: *When my boyfriend took me to his yoga class, I couldn't hold it together and burst out laughing and had to leave the class. We ended up having a big fight afterward. Honestly, it was easier to laugh at everyone than to dive into the whole yoga thing and figure out what it was all about—how it might be good for me even. But hey, yoga is a bit like music, right? There are lots of styles, and I am into some styles and not others.*

Does your body feel more like an enemy than a friend?

LING: *When I first started the Body Scan, I just wanted to fidget. No, it was worse than that: I just wanted to scream and run away.*

If you start with an especially difficult relationship with your body, you may get discouraged, feeling like you have too far to go to be truly comfortable with your body or every part of it. In this case, take it slow. Be gentle and supportive of yourself, simply acknowledging your urge to flee during practice as thoughts from a mind that wants you to flee. Mindfulness teachers can be a big help (our website signposts teachers offering classes).

Exploring the body with mindfulness can uncover the ways in which pain, historical emotional patterns, and trauma are embedded in the body. Sometimes we can register numbness or areas of pain that seem to have little to do with what's happening right now. When this happens, we can step back and say "No, not now," and we can move our attention elsewhere. In this way awareness is protective. Or we can choose to lean into these areas with kindly attention and care. Over time this can help them begin to come to life and loosen.

Dwelling on your expectations. We like quick results and get frustrated when they don't come. If your impatient response to doing the body-focused practices is that "this is not working," see if you can let go of your expectations. This isn't like strength training, where you expect to see your body changing session by session. It's more like planting a seed and seeing what grows. Yes, you need to water it and ensure it has the right amount of light, but poking around in the soil will halt its growth. Just get out of the way and let it teach you what it has to teach you!

> When learning a new mindfulness skill, focus on your intentions, not your expectations.

Inhabiting Your Body in Real Life, for the Rest of Your Life

SOPHIA (on her experience of a body-based mindfulness practice): *Breathing in, I can feel my belly rising, now it's falling, breathing out, now it's rising, I can feel my clothes and belt on my belly, there's some pressure, it changes with the inbreath and outbreath, it's a bit uncomfortable and tight. I need to weigh myself. Have I put on weight? I hope not, but I have been snacking too much in the evenings. I must stop buying peanut butter—I can't resist eating spoonfuls, yummy crunchy, oily dollops straight out of the jar. (Smiling) My dad used to do the same thing, I can see him now. My partner gave me a funny look the first time he saw me do this, ha, he doesn't anymore, he takes me as I am or he can find someone else. Mind wandering alert! Where was I, ah, my torso and my chest, I can feel my heart beating, almost like I can hear it, and feel a slight sense of blood pumping. Wow, that's pretty amazing. Is that real or am I imagining that? Now I can sense the pulsing, it's slow and steady, it's nice. Wow, I love this. And the breath alongside it in my chest, rising and falling. It's so still as I stand back and sense my breath and heartbeat. It's a bit like a snow globe, all the sediment is settling. Breathing in—beat, beat, breathing out, beat, beat, beat . . . wow. I feel really peaceful right now. Just at ease, it feels good. I wonder what time it is. Ah, my mind just wandered (smiling again), coming back, breathing in. . . . Sense of ease, connection, being at one with my body, mind, and life. Today, I am going to bring myself back throughout the day to this sense of being present in my body and keep anchoring myself. Including the tricky phone call I have to have with my friend today, I love her and want to put things right with her. My heart is beating a bit faster now, but I feel full of love. I've got this. Bring the day on.*

This is Sophia's experience of a mindfulness practice recently, attending to the breath and sensations in the body, the mind wandering (yes, she loves crunchy peanut butter and eats it by the spoonful out of the jar), being escorted back, sensing and wandering again, being interested in the different body states and sensations that come up, and inevitably come and go, with a sense of interest, even awe, thoughts about the day ahead, being able to gather and settle her awareness in her body. Remember practice is for life, and life is where the rubber hits the road. What comes up in Sophia's practice prepares her for the day ahead; she can draw on her practice to steady her and point her in the right direction throughout her day.

"I can't believe what I said to my friend yesterday. It was so thoughtless. I could see she was hurt. I need, no want, to apologize—I will call her today."

"Sometimes with my partner, I feel judged. And being able to accept each other as we are is something we're working on."

These are examples of where practice and life come together. If you can bring your mindfulness practice to your everyday life, then you're starting to live your life in a way that is more aligned with who you are and who you want to be, with how you want your life to be. You are choosing to recognize, allow, and savor the good moments.

This practice is for life, and the more you integrate it, the more it becomes second nature, even in the most challenging of situations. What happens when the body that has become a familiar, trustworthy, protective friend seems to turn on us through illness or age? Can you keep coming home to your body during a really busy period, when the demands on you require steadiness, good judgment, and your very best problem solving? For all of us, how do we respond to falling in love, to losing love, pregnancy, parenting, middle age, and retirement? This is the real *real* that we're dealing with—and, if we're lucky, will be dealing with for years to come. How can we keep inhabiting our body to meet all the inevitable changes and challenges in our lives?

Keeping the Body in Mind: The 50–50 Practice

The 50–50 practice is one that people find one of the most useful in mindfulness for life because it is a way of keeping your body in mind, as an anchor, teacher, and guide, throughout your day, whatever you are doing. It helps you to pay attention to whatever you're doing (50% of your awareness) and keep some of your awareness in your body (the other 50%). In this way your body can serve as an anchor. Whatever is happening, it can help you tune in to the "climate" of a given moment—calm, heated; safe, unsafe. In this way it acts as a guide. You can use both experiential and thinking modes of mind, listening to what each is telling you. In this way it acts as a teacher, so you can be more deliberate in your life.

PRACTICE: 50-50

You can follow along on our website.

You have practiced intentionally bringing awareness to physical sensations during the Body Scan practice and in everyday life. The 50-50 practice brings the two together. You give 50% of your attention to your body and 50% to whatever you're doing. You might start by trying it when you're talking to someone. As you are talking to this person, choose anywhere in the body that works for you, ideally somewhere that in that moment feels available to anchor your attention. This might be the sensations of contact between feet and floor, the sensations of sitting, the feel of the hands, and the sensations of breathing. And alongside this, give 50% of your attention to the person you're with, what they're saying, not just their words, but their nonverbal communication as well. See if you can keep track of these two parts of your awareness, what's happening with the other person and what's happening in your body. Your body is an anchor, but also a teacher and a guide.

   Next hold in mind both whatever you're doing and whatever is happening in the anchor in your body.

SOPHIA: *So I called my friend to apologize for my thoughtless comment yesterday. As I was about to call, I felt quite uptight, my breathing was shallow, and I was clammy—I was nervous. I anchored myself in my feet and did some stretches bringing her to mind, reminding myself how much I value her friendship and her happiness. I decided to stay standing as I called, by the window looking out at the trees in my garden. When she picked up, I felt an immediate connection; we've known each other since we were kids, and warmth spreading through me, even though these was still some fear in my chest. As we chatted, I tried to let go of my fear, because that was all about me, and see if I could apologize from the love. She was, as ever, so gracious in accepting my apology—she had felt hurt—and I noticed the fear melting and the sense of love spreading through my torso, arms, hands, neck, and head. After the call, I had a sense of being like the trees I was looking at in my garden, rooted, strong, swaying unfazed in the breeze.*

   Notice that Sophia didn't get fixed on whether her attention was divided evenly. The key is to have some sense of your ratio of thinking to experiencing as you go about your life—it can be 80–20, 40–60; any balance is useful. You'll lose that balance, forget to do the practice, lose track of your intention to do it. Don't worry about that either; the moment of knowing you are lost is part of the learning. That moment may take seconds or minutes, or it could be hours, or even days and weeks!

> Your body isn't going anywhere; it is always there, ready to come home to, to teach you and guide you.

How else could you use the 50–50 practice?

- When you go online—videoconferencing, checking social media, playing a game—do you start to feel tired, a bit disconnected, or unreal? Try anchoring yourself in the 50–50 practice to see what you notice in your body and mind. Do you learn anything that changes this experience? Or that changes how much time you spend online and in what ways?

- When you make a transition from one activity to another or one environment to another, do you ever find yourself ill at ease? I remember that moment when every summer I returned from my vacation and came back to work and switched my computer on for the first time. Why did I feel so fidgety when I had just had a really good time away from my job? When I started to do this with 50–50 awareness, I found I was returning to work with a sense of fear—what problems would I discover?—and dread: how many hundreds of emails and tasks would need doing? I am very lucky to have a job that I mostly love. So I shifted quite intentionally to reminding myself why I love my job and holding this attitude in mind as I made the transition from vacation to work. It had quite a radical effect. I still had the thoughts "I wonder what problems I will discover and how many tasks there will be to do." But the 50–50 practice added lots of other elements to the mix: "I wonder how my colleagues are getting on. Which projects am I most looking forward to this year? It will be good to reconnect with some of my closest collaborators."

- When in crisis or going through an unanticipated change, do you find yourself returning to old habits of 100% thinking?

> MOHAMMED: *This year Eid al-Fitr, when my family breaks its fast at the end of Ramadan, was different. I was really aware of what happened in my body with fasting during daylight and how it affected everything, my energy, my libido, my sense of being cleansed and healthy. My parents are from a different generation, my father is obese and so is my mother, she has diabetes as well, so Eid in our family was a bit of a gluttonous blowout. My wife and I talked about changing how we as a family eat, what we eat and when we eat, listening to what our body is telling us is right. It's helped us become much more intentional about our eating; lessons I hope our kids will also take forward.*

- Are your relationships ever a source of stress, reactivity, or worry? Of course they are. They are for everyone at various points in time. To find out how the 50–50 practice might illuminate what's going on and what you could do about it, consider starting simply, with someone with whom you have an easy relationship, doing something very neutral. This could be a parent checking on their sleeping child, sitting with a partner watching TV, playing video games with friends online. Bring some of your attention to your body. What do you notice? Does it change how you are with this person? Then maybe work up to more charged relationships, maybe a relationship with a colleague or friend that can be tricky, and situations, a difficult conversation or even conflict. Again, when you anchor yourself in this way, what do you notice? Your body is telling you important stuff that you can use going forward, *for life*.

SOPHIA: *The first time my partner "caught me" eating peanut butter out of the jar, we were watching TV and during a commercial break I had gone into the kitchen for my snack. He looked over his shoulder at me and in that moment my body was powerfully telling me something: I felt this shrinking feeling, horror, shame, judged. I could have just swallowed it, but I took a moment and had a little word with myself—"In my own home I can do as I please—eat what I like, when I like, how I like." We talked about it, and I realized he has a touch of OCD about hygiene—that was what his look was mostly about, his fear of germs. So now we have two peanut butter jars, his and hers. And understanding each other better helps us take care of each other better.*

What about our relationship with the wider world and all the issues that affect us—education, health care, our neighborhood, and country. We affect and are affected by the metaphorical and literal climate we live in. Here too the 50–50 practice can be our anchor, guide, and teacher.

SAM: *I am not big on watching the news, seems kind of pointless, because there's nothing I can do about it. But then my hospital had a series of power outages last year. The backup generators even failed one time. Couldn't ignore it anymore—it had to do with climate change and the strain on the power grid. Being in an ICU without power and air conditioning is downright scary. We lost one patient without the ventilators one time. It made me feel so angry and helpless—like I was stuck in quicksand. For my sanity, as much as anything, I had to do something. I got on board with this group that looks at local ways we can make a difference, downloaded an app that's helped me reduce my carbon footprint—bike rather than car, train rather than plane, and locally farmed vegetables and no red meat. I don't know how much difference I'm making, but at least I feel like I'm doing something.*

Connecting with Others throughout Life

Whether it's through gaze, touch, hugging, or physical intimacy, we use our bodies to connect with others in many ways that don't involve words. Obviously, the body is involved in all of our relationships, both transitory and enduring. Still, we sometimes *don't* stay connected to our bodies as we connect with others throughout our day. How do our interactions go if we're *not* connected to our bodies? How do we respond to the people around us as we go about our day? How do they respond to us if we're not aware of the body language we're using when we encounter them? Can we offer a touch to reassure someone who is struggling? Can we adopt a look that asserts our strength in the face of bullying behavior? Will we hug a loved one we haven't seen for a while? Can we act wisely on our sexuality?

PRACTICE: Connecting with Ourselves, Connecting with Others

You can follow along on our website.

This everyday practice can be used in moments of human connection, be that a smile, a hug, or an embrace. In the moments before you come into contact, follow your breathing and establish a sense of presence in your body. As you come into contact with the other person, have a real sense of them, using whatever senses are appropriate—seeing, listening, smelling, touching. Stay in contact with your breath and body and the resonance of connection in each moment. Can you have a *real sense of them*, connecting with all your body, mind, and heart? Can you widen this sense of yourself, the other person, and your connection in this moment? In the look, touch, or embrace, can you hold your own and one another's wholeness?

   Intention is key. This involves being open to your own and the other person's presence. Can you lightly ask the question, "What will serve your and the other person's well-being?" In these moments you, the other person, and the space between you come to life and are full of possibility.

> MOHAMMED: *I love watching people being reunited at airports, train, and bus stations. The moments when loved ones see each other again after being separated, the connection that comes from a smile, a hug, or a kiss. It lights me up. My brother visited recently, and we have at times had a strained relationship. In the moment we hugged hello at the airport, I said to myself under my breath, "Here he is, here we are, he smells so familiar. It's good to have him here. I want us to reset, to put our differences behind us and bring all that is good forward and build on that—we're brothers after all."*

The Ancient Oak: Intra-being and Inter-being

The Vietnamese monk Thich Nhat Hahn coined the terms *intra-* and *inter-being* to remind us that we can be aware of our minds and bodies (intra-being), but if we really open up to others, our awareness expands to include a realm of being in relationship with others (inter-being). Actually, he extended this to the wider world, and in a letter to the United Nations said, "The Earth is not something outside of us. Breathing with mindfulness and contemplating your body, you realize that you are the Earth. You realize that your consciousness is also the consciousness of the Earth. Look around you—what you see is not your environment, it is you."

It takes courage to be open, to let ourselves be seen fully, not just by others but by ourselves—our strength and vulnerability, our potential for both generosity and mean-spiritedness, not just our good side, but also the parts of ourselves we tend to hide away.

SOPHIA: *When I started out as a teacher, I dreaded kids making inappropriate, sexist, and mean comments to one another and to me. It took a few years to become a more embodied teacher, owning my power. I could teach from a place where the kids knew the boundaries and knew I would uphold them. My classroom became safe, and we could get to the business of learning.*

SAM: *When I first started having sex, I was a bundle of nerves. First off, there was the whole deal of how I felt about my own body—skinny Sam. But the real problem was that everything I knew about sex I had learned through porn or the slightly awkward talks with a high school friend who was a few years ahead of me in his explorations. Needless to say, this wasn't the best crash course. My first escapades felt like I was starring in some awkward porn video, where I was the actor, director, filmmaker, and entire audience. Terrible. It took me ages to let go of thinking what sex should be like, what I should be like. I had to ditch the whole actor, director, filmmaker, and audience mindset. Only then could I start enjoying being in my own body and with the guys I was exploring with, enjoying each other.*

Connecting with others and the wider world reminds us that we are not islands. This is the basis for understanding, real dialogue, connection, sexuality, reconciliation, and managing all the moments in the natural life course of any relationship.

Cultivating Wisdom through Our Bodies

Your body will tell you things your mind will talk you out of.
Your body is telling you what direction life is in. Try trusting it.
                                                    —GLENNON DOYLE

Your body can be a wise teacher. It has been learning throughout your life and, much more than this, throughout evolution, how to alert and orient us to important information about safety, connection, satiety, energy, health. Attending to what is happening in your body and mind can yield all sorts of helpful insights.

LING: *When I was first with the father of my children, we were soulmates. I felt safe with him. I felt I could turn off my constant high alert. Sex felt like two people really connecting. He always had my back. I remember once I was in trouble with not being able to make rent one month—I was on edge, constantly worrying, "would I be asked to move out," "where would I go, what would happen to my kids?" He paid the rent, no note, no expectation of paying him back. His generosity, with his time, support, and financially, was like a drug, making me feel safe and cared for; I'd never had that before.*

But over time I noticed that I started to not feel good around him, jittery. It started with small things, he'd say—"Sure, you can go to the gym, but I'll be lonely home alone." Then he started with being openly critical— "You're selfish; that gym membership is money you could use to pay your rent." A pattern of low-level criticism and control set into our relationship that left me feeling bad about myself and guilty about my needs. Sex became less about connection and more about his needs. It made me snarky with him too, and I didn't want to have sex with him anymore. But he was also a good dad, mostly, and could be funny and charming. He could disarm me with a look or a word.

I spoke to my friends—they all gave different advice. I joined an online forum for women, but while the people were trying to be helpful, they were talking about themselves, what had worked, or not, for them. Lots of people were hurt and angry. I let go of analyzing the situation and paid attention to what came up in my body in my mindfulness practice over several months. I realized that my being on high alert and fear were back—I didn't feel safe anymore. In the middle of practices, when my mind was very settled, I'd sometimes ask questions and see what bubbled up, if anything. Questions like "What would support my well-being, my kids' well-being, his well-being?" "What is the kind of relationship that I want?" "What kind of life do I want?" "Does this situation enlarge or diminish me?" Instead of trying to answer the questions, I simply let the questions drop into my practice and then experience my mind and body. I noticed that things felt out of kilter, not right, that I longed to be safe, to be somewhere where I was free from relentless criticism and control, where I could expand and be myself. And I felt scared. Yes, he had always had my back in a way no one else ever had. But I realized with a chill running down my spine that I'd become scared of him. It took some months, but this practice helped me realize that my relationship had to change radically, and if it couldn't, I had to leave.

I've seen people I love go through childbirth, menopause, illness, and I've seen several people go through the final months of life as their bodies closed down as they moved toward death. I've made some major decisions in my life, sometimes decisions that involved loss, pain, and hurt. The body guides us through the major passages in life and leads us to these important decisions.

Coming Home to Your Body for Life

I have heard this joke more than once. "Why do professors have a body? To move their brains from the lecture hall to the library, to the laboratory." Whatever your vocation or profession, you may identify with this idea that your brain is everything and your body is simply a vehicle to carry your brain around. But when we know our body as our body, contemplate the changing nature of our body, consider the body free from the wish for it to be different from what it is, and contemplate the common humanity and universal story of all bodies, we can see the power of mindfulness for life. Our bodies are with us from the moment we're born to the moment we die—for better or worse, in sickness and in health. For as long as we're alive, there's almost certainly more right with our bodies than wrong, so why not befriend and really inhabit your body? If you can come to know and trust your body, it becomes like coming home, or perhaps even realizing you were already home but didn't know it. This idea of living with appreciation is what we turn to next.

4

Appreciating the Life We Have

Find the beauty in the muddle
—ANONYMOUS

A friend of mine is a nurse with years of experience in palliative care. Her patients are often in considerable distress—understandable as they typically have less than a year to live. Whenever she talks about her work, she radiates light and compassion. In fact, to me it seems that her whole life is filled with joy; she always has time for friends, adventure, and fun. She laughs a lot. This in spite of the fact that I know she's encountered more than her fair share of life's challenges. And like all of us, she can have good days and bad days. My overriding sense of her is that she lives her life with a real sense of *carpe diem*. As a psychologist I tend to ask quite direct questions, so I asked her: "How do you find so much joy in your life? How do you stay full of compassion, having seen so much suffering in your work?" Without missing a beat, she responded, "I find the beauty in the muddle."

How many times throughout the day do you miss moments of beauty, joy, and fun? You can be so busy muddling through life that you miss out on these moments. Or perhaps you just skate over them because you're on autopilot or moving through your day at double speed, taking care of all the have-to-dos of life. Or perhaps your mind is set up somehow to orient to everything other than joy.

Think back over a typical day. How often do you have a sense of "the beauty in the muddle"? How often do you feel a sense of joy? When you do, are you able to stop to savor these moments? Moments of happiness, friendship, gratitude, fun, the sense of achievement at getting something done, the pleasure of seeing someone you care about doing well, moments of seeing beauty in nature? Waking up to see today's weather, and to accept and appreciate it for what it is, the ever-changing weather and seasons? Can you pause and appreciate these moments?

> MOHAMMED: *Parenting is exhausting; it can be relentless. I often feel like I have lost my life. But there are some moments every day when the kids are so adorable, when they say cute stuff, or when they're asleep and my daughter can look like an angel—she isn't (laughing). These moments sort of charge my battery for the rest of the day. And you know I do have some moments, when my wife gives them a bath in the evening, the minutes before I fall asleep, which I have started to really appreciate.*

The idea of paying attention was introduced in Chapter 2. In Chapter 3 you saw how the body can be an anchor, sanctuary, and guide. But this is only the start of the story. You can, with applied effort, cultivate attitudes of mind. As my nurse friend exemplified, it's possible to remain happy, optimistic, and positive in the midst of working with pain, suffering, and death. What was her secret?

"Look for the Good"

Alice Herz-Sommer, a World War II survivor of Auschwitz, went on to lead a happy life well into old age. At 106, when an interviewer asked her, "What is your secret?" she said. "Look for the good" and "Be thankful." Then she said something important: "I know about the bad things, but I look for the good things." She had seen humanity's darkest side and was coping with failing health and approaching death, yet this remained the message she wanted to pass on.

Looking for the good in the face of the bad things in life. The perpetuation of our species demanded that we pay immediate attention to threats to our survival. In evolutionary terms, in fact, there is no obvious need for joy or happiness. Even our extraordinary capacity for thinking and communication evolved for other reasons—planning, learning from experience, social and community cohesion. So it's only natural, even today, that we can easily overlook experiences that are enjoyable, rewarding, and give us a sense of purpose. Alice Herz-Sommer is describing a choice to bring a certain innocence of perception and an orientation to the good, which she has cultivated throughout her life. We know from research with experienced meditators that this is something we can learn and develop, and when we do it is associated with well-being.

People who experience recurrent depression often say that recovery is not just about tackling depression; it is also about learning what it takes to stay well and enjoy a high quality of life. Barney Dunn, a professor of clinical psychology at the University of Exeter, has found that well-established psychological therapies that help people learn to respond to negative thoughts and get back to being active are not sufficient to help people recover from depression. They also need to learn what is enjoyable and meaningful to them and then spend more time on these activities. As one person who suffers from depression put it, it's not just about learning to turn away from the dark, but also about learning to live in the light.

Cultivating Joyfulness

The tree which moves some to tears of joy is in the eyes
of others only a green thing which stands in the way.
—WILLIAM BLAKE

So what can we learn from the people who've experienced horrors and from modern research? It takes only a small step out of habit and into awareness to enjoy the people we love around us, to savor food, or to dance to music in our kitchen while cooking. These moments are available to us all the time if we choose to attend to them and, more than that, enjoy them. Joy is not about sentimentality or over-the-top excitement. When we're carried away by the *idea* of joy, making it something to think and talk about, rather than living it, we lose contact with these joyful states of mind and body—gladness, energy, love, contentment, wonder, radiant pride, delight, beauty, and gratitude.

> What joyful states are important to you?

You can explore these states with beginner's mind again, perhaps as you did when you experienced them for the first time, before they became habitual or defined as "not new or interesting" and so not worth attending to. The way a strawberry tasted the first time you tasted one, the way you felt the first time you fell in love, or the way as a young person you felt safe and happy with your first best friend or pet. *Joy has its roots in this wholehearted appreciative attention, this innocence of perception, this beginner's mind.*

PRACTICE: Three-Step Breathing Space Revisited

Appreciation can be unfamiliar and a new skill, so you may need some support to integrate it into your life. The Three-Step Breathing Space (see Chapter 3, page 60) is a way to pause, anchor, and then open. If you are going into a situation that you know you will enjoy, take a Breathing Space just before. This will help you.

SAM: *I dove in to bike road racing, and before kicking off I also do a Breathing Space. It gets me in sync; last time out I was so pumped up for the ride. During the ride I check in, soaking it all in. It makes it all super vivid and rich. It's a real game-changer being—being in flow when I ride—there is always a whole mix of stuff happening, good, bad, and everything in between. Riding isn't all sunshine—there's quite a lot of pain too, especially on the intense hills. Man, that feeling of relief at the top is sweet. Then there are the downhills; exhilarating, sure, but as day follows night, an incline follows a downhill.*

PRACTICE: Appreciating the Life You Have, Each Day

You can follow along on our website.

As you go about your day, make a habit of seeing, touching, and listening wholeheart-edly, aware of how you are touching and being touched by the world. Take moments to pause. Feel the warmth of the sun, the breeze on your skin. See not only the trees but also the space around the trees; not only the stars but also the vastness of the sky that holds the stars. Sense the small moments of generosity you extend to or receive from others—the smile, the door held open. Hear the laughter of a child on the playground. Fully taste the food you eat. Reflect on all that goes well for you today—your ability to move through the world, to be fed and warm, and to care for yourself. In every moment, sense what it is that holds the potential to gladden your heart when you are truly present.

Each day, intentionally bring awareness to something that you do regularly and know you enjoy. It could be anything: a morning cup of tea or coffee, a walk, a favorite snack, an interaction with someone you appreciate or love, a person or a pet, or a spa-cious moment in your day while you travel. Commit to being wholeheartedly present, aware of your bodily sensations, feelings, and thoughts. Bring an innocent perception and sensitivity to the experience. Explore each of the senses in turn: seeing, hear-ing, taste, touch, smell. Really sense how attention imbued with innocent perception affects your experience of this moment. Allow your heart to tremble in the midst of the experience, gladdened by the simplicity of the moment.

LING: *I was swimming and floating in a friend's pond recently, and because I had just learned this practice, I was able to be more fully aware of the beauty of the moment. The feel of myself immersed in the water, mostly warm, but with some colder patches, the smell of pine resin, the sounds of laughter, the warm glow of friendship, her dog lying on the shore desperate to join in. I turned to her, smiled, and said, "This is a good moment." She met my eye, smiled back, and said simply, "Yes, yes it is."*

TROUBLESHOOTING: Getting Out of Our Own Way to Cultivate Joy

When you recover or discover something that
nourishes your soul and brings joy, care enough
about yourself to make room for it in your life.
—JEAN SHINODA BOLEN

You need to make room for cultivating appreciation, joy, and gratitude—form
the intention, make the time, and put in the work. But it's not easy, especially
when we have full and challenging lives or have learned to approach our lives
with a mindset of striving and judging. Some of us have picked up beliefs like
"I can barely hold things together—now you want me to do this? Instead of my
commitments? No way." These beliefs can generate feelings of guilt, anger, even
shame. They turn us away from appreciation and joy.

But what you'll learn is that joy inspires you to practice more, because
it feels good, you learn from it, and it resources you. Even when you're busy,
perhaps especially when you're really busy, you can start to find moments to lift
your gaze and open up to good moments—when you learn that this can help
you with the busyness, you want to do it because you know it not only feels
good but helps you get through these times too.

*What is the difference between healthy savoring (I guess noticing it when
it comes) and unhelpful craving/wanting (I guess chasing it)?* You might think
of it as a continuum. Laying a little bit of the groundwork to give you the best
chance of pleasure coming is helpful, while setting very high, rigid expectations
of where that will take you is problematic.

Our judging and striving mind skates over or avoids moments of joy. As
you've already seen, our unhappiness can stem from our judging mind, where
you forever see the gap between how things are and how you think they ought
to be. This is solidified by the stories you create. An example is believing that
our happiness depends on having the same successes and possessions as others.
When you do get some of these possessions, you have a moment of happiness,
only to find it slipping away once more as other gaps appear between how you
think things should be and how you feel they are. At school and work, grades
and performance reviews serve to feed our sense of inadequacy. They only
strengthen our tendency to be the person we feel we should be. It's like a thirst
that no amount of water can quench. We mistake it for the pursuit of joy. But
it disconnects us from our values, appreciative joy, and the possibility of lasting
contentment. Rather than look for joy within what we already have, we make

it about owning things, achieving things, and reaching endless goals. Stepping off this hamster wheel and letting go of the impulse of compulsive wanting enables us to connect with our intentions, step into appreciative joy, and cultivate the conditions for a more stable contentment.

For people living with depression, anxiety, chronic pain, and illness, the absence of gladness leads the mind to become increasingly despairing and bleak. Anxiety and depression leach joy out of our lives. Joy becomes a distant memory or a faint prospect. Our world shrinks, until difficulty is the only thing we can see. Overcoming depression is about learning how our habits of mind and body can sometimes trip us up in seeing and approaching the light. And learning to notice this and continuing to move toward the glimmer rather than getting lost in the dark.

> LING: *I was coming out of a difficult time in my life. I'd been quite low and tired—no particular reason, just being a single parent to teenage kids, working, juggling everything. I have become more and more prone to these periods of being low. When I first tried these appreciation exercises, nothing much came up. My life's just not been great recently. It was like putting a search term into Google and no results coming up. But at the bottom it suggests other search terms, so I stuck with it and tried those search terms instead. I realized my daughter had been really trying, the TV series I am watching in the evenings makes me laugh, at lunch at work I have been going out for walks with a colleague—when we get back, I realize I feel good. There have been some small things keeping me afloat. I tried paying more attention to these moments and making it an active choice to take these walks and do things that made me laugh.*

It takes only a simple intention and a moment of mindfulness amid difficulty, pain, or illness to notice the places in your body that are well. Gladness is not a reward for having endured or survived the difficult—rather, it is one of the key qualities that allows us to embrace the difficult without being overwhelmed by it and to appreciate all that is good. In any given moment, you can steady the mind and orient to joy, one breath at a time. The key to contentment is seeing and letting go of the relentless judging mind and instead resting in our experience exactly as it is. It can be helpful to ask, "What do I need in this moment to be happy?" "What is missing from this moment?" The expression "You're as happy as you make up our minds to be" also suggests this deliberate intention and action of mind to both reclaim and cultivate joy.

> SOPHIA: *When I first retired, somehow I was just as busy as ever. How did that happen? The busyness was not something I enjoyed; it crowded the joy out of my days. I*

*needed the ten-finger appreciation practice (see Chapter 1, page 17) to remind me what
was important to me. I had to learn to notice and let go of the judgmental thoughts, like
"I don't deserve to be happy."*

It is easy to get in our own way. When people say to me, "I tried mindfulness, but it wasn't for me," I am really curious. I wonder what they mean first
by "mindfulness" and then by "I tried mindfulness." If we focus on the breath,
body, or our actions in a rather cold way, paying attention is like a "blank
stare." Over time we will lose interest. It can even bring a harsh, judgmental,
striving attitude to mindfulness practice. We may find ourselves cajoling, giving ourselves a hard time—"It's not good enough . . . I'm a failure at this. . . .
If only I could get this right." The mindfulness practice becomes like a boot
camp—"I must try harder; I'm not working hard enough." Over time these attitudes will more than likely make mindfulness practice aversive. Appreciation
means stepping away from habit, especially those that shut down joy or throw
a veil in the way of contentment. Strange as it may sound, this takes practice;
it is a skill to be learned and honed.

Broadening and Building Appreciation and Joy into Your Life, for Life

How can you build appreciation into life, for life?

SOPHIA: *A few years into retirement I started to keep a diary on my bedside table, and
each day I jotted down what I appreciated from the day. One New Year's Eve, I read
back through all the entries and some themes came up again and again. Making gifts
for people I really care about, using my writing and craft skills. Taking care of Noah,
my grandson. My dog Rufus, walking him every day, his friendship and loyalty. Meeting my boyfriend and getting to know each other, the growing intimacy and connection
of physical intimacy, which if I'm honest I've missed so much since my husband died.
Cooking, especially for other people. Taking a nap in the reclining lounger in my back
garden in the sun . . . waking up and feeling a glow of being refreshed by a daytime
nap. So, my New Year's resolution was to build these into my days and weeks—to
make them a central part of the fabric of my life. I know what you're thinking, New
Year's resolutions don't work. But you'd be wrong here because it wasn't difficult. Who
couldn't want to do things that bring joy into their life?*

Appreciation is neither a checklist nor a thinking exercise. Instead, it is a deliberate practice in the spirit of living with a sense of *carpe diem*, both in the small moments of the day and in the more substantive moments of our lives. What does this mean? It means noting how our bodies are in these moments, what moods and emotions are around, what thoughts and images come up. This is how you turn good things into good experiences.

Like a gardener tending a garden over years, you can cultivate this appreciative attitude of mind. As with gardening, when you put in effort, nature sort of takes over. It takes time, sometimes a whole season or even several seasons. This is what Sophia is doing, cultivating appreciation and joy by seeing patterns in her life, doing more of what she knows will create the right conditions for joy and then getting out of her own way.

If you look back at your appreciation practice, which are the most recurrent themes? What are the top five most frequent people, places, things, or experiences that in the last week, month, year brought you a sense of joy? How would it be to deliberately schedule these into your life? This involves going from noticing what you appreciate to intentionally integrating these into your life. This can be a lifelong practice, and the themes will likely change at different stages of your life. For Sophia, in the example above, it was her dog, her grandson Noah, her new boyfriend Chris, being in touch with her children and taking time in her kitchen for the first cup of tea of the day. For people who are working, or who have children, or who are studying the themes will likely be different.

Dance as If No One Is Watching

I love the expression "Dance as if no one is watching." It gets at our tendency to constantly judge ourselves and others, which can be paralyzing. This is especially true in England, where the stereotype of being rather "buttoned up" can get in the way of letting go and enjoying ourselves. When my daughters were teenagers, they were mortified if they came into the kitchen to find me listening to music and dancing while cooking. They never believed me when I said I did this even if I was home alone. Of course, the wider point is that as you learn this attitude of mind, you can start to do what brings joy into your life without letting judgment imprison us.

> What are your top five sources of joy? How would it be to schedule these into your life?
>
> What gets in the way of prioritizing joy? What would it be like if you did, and joy became an integral part of your life?

The Barefoot Professor: Music and Dance in Human Evolution

Professor Robin Dunbar at the University of Oxford, who studies psychology and evolution, has come up with some interesting theories about how music and dance were involved in the evolution of *Homo sapiens*. Dance and music, he suggests, probably predate our ability to communicate through language. They were a way of forming family bonds, as was grooming one another, but in the case of singing and dancing a whole group could do it together, enabling larger units to form, bond, and communicate before they had more fully developed language. Today anthropologists have shown that in some cultures dance is integral to how people interact—Brazil, to name one good example. There is more and more evidence that dancing and singing can support mental health and well-being. In some places it's being integrated into what's called "social prescribing," where various health and public health professionals "prescribe" these activities because they help us connect and make us feel better. We're coming full circle, prescribing what our *Homo sapiens* ancestors knew thousands of years ago was good, not only for themselves but also for their family.

> What could you do with all-out joy as if no one is watching?

As you become more aware of what brings us joy, what's important to you, you're at a crossroads. Do you take the risk to do more of what brings us joy and to "dance as if no one is watching"?

MOHAMMED: *As a student I worked hard to please my coach, teammates, and parents. I was always striving to be the best, on the sports ground, in the gym, my diet, weight—it was 24/7. When my injury ended my sports career, it was devastating. But people weren't watching me anymore, and honestly, it was a relief. I started, tentatively at first, to learn what I enjoyed and realized that going out, listening to music and dancing was a lot of fun. I loved dancing at the front of live gigs and didn't care what people thought—I was having a good time. I bought a great music system, and often I'd crank up the volume and dance as if no one was watching.*

A New Way of Being: Contentment

Over time transient moments of appreciation can become an abiding sense of contentment. A sense that all is well, that you can rest in this moment, where it's pleasant or unpleasant, with a sense of ease. A key to contentment is letting go of always judging everything—"if only, I ought to, I should, I need, I want, others should, others need, I am not good enough, it's not good enough, they're not good enough, when this or that happens, then. . . . " Judging, judging, judging. It's exhausting. You start to recognize when the judging mind kicks in, "Ah, here's the judge again." In these moments, with a sense of friendliness and care, you can let the judgments go. When you do, you choose to *rest* in your experience, pleasant, unpleasant, or neutral, *exactly as it is*. This question can be helpful:

"Is there anything I need <u>in this moment</u> to be happy? Is there anything lacking <u>in this moment?</u>"

This question can be a great teacher, exposing the judge and the way it triggers questions about our life, who we are, how we think things should be, how our mind can create a sense of lack. When you see the judge, and let it go, you can rest in your experience exactly as it is. To be clear, judging can be tremendously helpful when used wisely. It's when it is our default way of being that it can disrupt a sense of ease and contentment. Nor is it some Pollyanna, think-positive nonsense. As we saw from my friend the palliative care nurse, we can find joy and contentment in the muddle, in the midst of the challenges of life. The question "What else do I need in this moment to be contented?" is about *this moment*—if you rest your awareness just in this moment, what do you find? Can you rest in a sense of ease regardless of what you find?

> MOHAMMED: *When I first did this exercise, my mind immediately went to all the ways my life should be better—a part-time job, more money, less pain, more help with my kids, more help around the house, better gym equipment, my sports team winning a tournament for the first time in a decade! I noticed my mind creating this sense of if only, and when I came back to this moment, my back was okay, a small amount of throbbing, but manageable, and the rest of my body felt good actually. I could rest in the movement of my breath in-out, and feel a sense of ease, even with this background noise of my mind chattering about all the things I needed to do. My thoughts were just part of the background of this moment, alongside the throbbing in my back, the sense of my feet solid on the ground, my chest as it rose and fell with my breath, and a background pulse of my heartbeat, steady and slow.*

Contentment opens our eyes to the goodness that sits alongside difficulty. Deep contentment involves letting go of the search for perfection and stability that simply don't exist. It persists even when we're living through difficult times. After she told me about some of the ways in which people die, I asked my palliative care friend whether, if she was terminally ill, she would choose euthanasia. She looked me in the eye and said without pausing, "No, because even in the midst of the awfulness of dying I can see in my patients and their family something very precious and beautiful. I wouldn't want to miss out on that."

Thankfulness

Whenever you want to cheer yourself, think of the qualities of
your fellows—the energy of one, for example, the decency of
another, the generosity of a third, some other merit of a fourth.
There is nothing so cheering as the stamp of virtues manifest
in the character of colleagues. . . . So, keep them ready to hand.
                                                    —MARCUS AURELIUS

The good things in our lives, things we can appreciate and be grateful for,
are already here. Thankfulness nourishes and supports appreciation and joy. It
is an active choice to identify all that we can be grateful for in our lives. It is
noticing and bringing an attitude of thankfulness to the many aspects of our
lives that are going well. This can be gratitude for seemingly trivial things, like
a moment of kindness a stranger shows us, or more seemingly profound things,
like a loving relationship, or our health.

Thankfulness is not sentimental, it's not denying that there are difficult
things in our life and the wider world, nor is it necessarily easy. It is a practice, raising your gaze, broadening your horizon, recognizing what you have
in your life to be thankful for and taking the time to develop this capacity for
thankfulness. This practice of cultivating an attitude of appreciation can be
transformative because you're learning to shift your attention and the way you
relate to your experience.

Cultivating Appreciation, Joy, Contentment, and Thankfulness for Life

Over time joy helps you befriend difficulties and meet suffering with balance
and care. When a friend has some good news, for example, you can allow
envy to arise and entertain it: "Why does he get to have this [e.g., sporting or
academic success, new car, new relationship]?" Or you can choose to step back
from the envy and celebrate your friend's happiness. Over time you develop
a greater ability to find joy in others' happiness and success. Joy can become
a natural, familiar way of being. When we're anxious, low, or tired, we naturally foreground everything that is bad and banish all that is good into the
background. Recognizing this begins to widen our attentional field, so we can
see obsession and rumination with some distance. Heartache, worry, and pain
don't have to exclude appreciation and gladness—they can coexist. Joy and
ease can be found even in the bleakest landscapes. Although you can't engineer

joy or gratitude just like that, you can learn how to make room for gladness, how to drop into joy and see what you are thankful for. This is not denial, but rather recognizing your natural biases to focus on the difficult instead of on all that is well.

> SOPHIA: *I see happiness like myriad different pieces of colored glass in a kaleidoscope. When my husband died, the colors in my life changed. My relationship with him was a single piece of colored glass forming the kaleidoscope of my life. It was an important piece in that time—it was the blue piece (my favorite color). It added so much to how I saw the world at that time, but when I found out he was unwell I started to realize it was borrowed time. I didn't know when it was going to be taken away, and that made me sad. But when it fell away, I learned to live with the green and the pink and the yellow, and eventually I found that the color cobalt could be shades of blue, green, and yellow colors in combination. I learned to see new patterns and new forms of beauty. I still think about his shade of blue, though . . . it will always be important to me . . .*

Appreciation, joy, and gratitude don't have to wait until everything seems to be going well. It may take time, but it is an attitude that you can start to cultivate both in any moment and through mindfulness practice. Integrating these practices into your life gradually shifts perspective in a remarkable way. Appreciative joy is much more than just a passing moment. It is a quality of mind and heart, a way of being, a place to come home to. These are attitudes that can be cultivated. Over time they mature into a more enduring contentment.

5

Our Most Important
Natural Resource

Our "Body–Mind"

"It's been a busy week; I feel exhausted.""I'm checking my phone
every few minutes to see if the message I sent has been answered."

"My strings got pulled at work again."

"I feel worried about all the issues in the world, and helpless to do
anything about them."

Can you relate to any of these statements? What about these?

"When I am with this person, I feel safe and inspired."

"Going out tonight, I feel buzzy, excited."

"Looking at this work I've done, I feel proud, swelling with pride
even."

"I love my pet. When I get home he is always pleased to see me."

"I've been sick, and this is the first day I feel well again. There
should be a word for this state of thankfulness and fragility."

These may seem like just small unremarkable moments. But they are the
building blocks of our day and our lives, and learning anything of value normally means starting with the basics. You've started to gather your attention
when your mind is scattered and focus on what's important and brings you joy.
You've started to inhabit your body more fully because it can be a sanctuary
and a teacher. You're cultivating curiosity and appreciation, attitudes of mind
that enrich you. In this chapter you'll explore how your mind and body are
your most important natural resource because from the moment you are born
to the moment you die, they are what you have to make sense of and navigate
your world.

If you're familiar with psychology or psychological therapies like cognitive therapy, much of what you'll read in this chapter will be familiar. If you're not, you may come back to this chapter again and again, because this chapter will give you a strong foundation for everything that follows.

The Ancient Oak and the Barefoot Professor: Descartes Was Wrong

Descartes was a 17th-century thinker who famously said, "Cogito, ergo sum" or "I think, therefore I am." His argument was that our minds are somehow beyond and distinct from our bodies. He even hypothesized that we had a gland, the pineal gland, where our mind and body interacted. But psychological science and neuroscience now clearly show us that our mind and body are totally interconnected. This will become clear throughout this chapter, and to sidestep Descartes's error I'll refer to "body–mind" from now on.

How do we make sense of the world? It all starts with the four building blocks that make up much of our experience—bodily sensations, emotions, impulses, and thoughts. How quickly we make connections among them! An emotion such as fear can trigger a thought ("Oh, this is going to go badly wrong"). A thought ("My friend looks preoccupied, not in a good way") can also trigger an emotion (such as concern). We jump to conclusions, sometimes rightly, sometimes wrongly, especially if we're stressed or tired. With mindful awareness we can see how the mind creates stories—about who we are and aren't, what we think of others, our views of the world. Some of these stories are like shooting stars, appearing and disappearing quickly, like a sneeze: "I'm worried about the meeting later today" or "This aches." Others become enduring constellations, habits, maybe even our "personality," "the kind of person we are," the story of our lives. We take our moment-by-moment experiences and turn them into "My life is a mess," "I've lost my mojo," or "I am the sort of person who gets anxious a lot."

When you start to see the mind's powerful ways of constructing reality, you can start to play an active part in this process.

Learning from the Body–Mind

I know of no more encouraging fact than the unquestionable ability of man (sic) to elevate his life by conscious endeavor. It is something to be able to paint a particular picture, or to carve a statue, and so to make a few objects beautiful; but it is far more glorious to carve and paint the very atmosphere and medium through which we look. . . . To affect the quality of the day, that is the highest of arts.

—HENRY DAVID THOREAU

How Our Senses Create Our Experience

You've already learned to slow everything down so you can see how each of your senses creates your experience in any moment. You've tried a mindfulness practice that involved simply seeing (Chapter 2). Let's try another sense, hearing.

PRACTICE: **Hearing**

You can follow along on our website.

In this practice you use your attention like a high-quality microphone. Your hearing, the microphone, registers all the sounds, coming and going, exactly as they are. You'll soon notice that your mind wants to give a sound a name or even a story—this is a car passing outside or the sound of my breath. This is a chance to note gently and firmly what's happening and bring yourself back, as best you can, to just hearing. It's the kind of microphone a professional sound engineer would use that can pick up all sounds well.

PRACTICE: **Hearing, Taking It Further**

You can follow along on our website.

You can extend the hearing practice by bringing in the idea of a sound engineer and a mixing desk. In this extension of the hearing practice, you're a sound engineer using the mixing desk to turn up some sounds, so some are in the foreground of awareness, and turn others down, so they fade into the background.

Your mixing desk also has filters. What I mean is you can transform your experience by dialing up the different attitudes you've started to explore. First, a childlike curiosity; a sense of "I've never heard this before." Perhaps an attitude of friendliness. Welcoming and befriending your experience. This is like using the mixing desk to add an ambient warmth to the experience of hearing.

Finally, you can open more of the channels on the mixing board so there is a sense of wider awareness, so all sounds, foreground and background, are in the field of hearing. This wider perspective also enables you to see in real time the way experience is continually created and re-created. See if you can recognize the moment a sound is registered, the moment it is registered as pleasant, unpleasant, or neutral, the moments you become aware of its qualities (pitch, volume, location in space), the way the mind so quickly and automatically gives each sound a name, sometimes even a story? Can you stand back, track each link in the chain as the mind does this amazing work of hearing—of making sense of sounds?

Our Different Senses

Everyone knows the classic five senses—seeing, hearing, tasting, smelling, and touching. Early philosophers, like Aristotle, were the first to speculate that smell could arise from particles emitted by plants and flowers and that these could have health benefits. These smells attract animals, bees, butterflies, birds, and bats, and this helps plant reproduction. The smell literally shapes their behavior. Since then, we've learned that smell is detected at the top of our nasal cavity in the olfactory epithelium, the size of a postage stamp, made of 4 million olfactory neurons. Smell involves receptors in areas of our nose binding with molecules in the air and sending signals through nerve endings to a part of the brain called the *olfactory bulb*, which via the olfactory cortex, just above it, is linked to many networks and areas throughout the brain that control what we do and how we feel. Professor Kathy Willis at the University of Oxford is a botanist who has looked at the research and concludes that there is a growing body of evidence showing that smells (cedar, citrus fruits) can have physiological (anti-inflammatory, anti-allergic) and psychological (soothing) benefits. Beyond seeing, hearing, tasting, and smell, we also sense touch, temperature, time, hunger/thirst, and balance. Think about how real this is when you experience extremes of hot/cold, are very hungry or thirsty, you've traveled across time zones and feel disoriented, or you have some condition like an ear infection that affects your sense of balance. All the senses together help us make sense of our world.

The Barefoot Professor: Perception and Cognition

Psychologists have discovered that seeing is not like a video camera and hearing is not like a microphone; it is much more like a production suite; all that we sense we touch up, fill in, and write stories based on all we've learned in our lives. . . . It is a creative process! Hearing involves pitch, volume, tone, patterns, but it also involves filling in the gaps and integrating it into a whole. One of the first psychologists, William James, put it this way: "The mind works on data it receives as a sculptor on a block of stone."

All our experience starts with our senses. Mindfulness helps us see the process of hearing, seeing, sensing what is happening in our bodies. I hope I have given you an idea of how awe inspiring our senses are and how they can serve you.

SAM: *I was on a first date. He was good looking, and I felt a chemistry right from the get-go. I can't describe it, but I felt it. When I saw he was smiling, not just with his mouth, but his eyes, all of him, I felt all aglow inside. When he touched my hand, obviously flirting now, I had a shot of electricity run through me. It was fun, I was happy. I relaxed and enjoyed myself.*

Learning to See How Our Thoughts Shape Our Reactions

Our thoughts powerfully shape our experience. Here is an example.

> LING: *So, I'm walking down the street and I see my friend on the other side. I smile and wave at her. She carries on walking. In that moment I feel terrible, just terrible, like I wish the sidewalk would just swallow me up.*

How did this scene unfold? Ling's friend kept walking without acknowledging her wave, and Ling felt terrible.

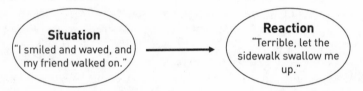

How would you have reacted in this situation? Perhaps something like this has happened to you? So here is the key question for Ling: What thoughts went through her mind when her friend kept walking?

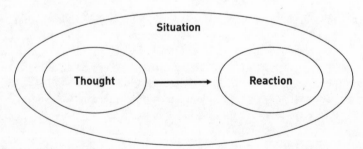

For Ling the thoughts were "I have upset her somehow—oh no, how embarrassing. I hope no one saw." When we see them written down like they are in the diagram, it makes sense of her reaction; we can see why she felt the way she did, why she wanted the sidewalk to swallow her up.

Ling was trying to make sense of her friend walking by without waving back.

This example shows how immediate our reactions can be. As you've already explored, this is because our mind is always anticipating "what's next" and setting us up to react based on these predictions. Using everything you've learned to date in how you react happens at every level, experientially in the body, but also in thinking, where memories, ideas, and the wider social context shape your reactions. The philosopher Jiddu Krishnamurti put it this way: "The day you teach the child the name of the bird, the child will never see that bird again." What he is saying is that the minute we call what we are seeing "a bird," we stop really seeing it or hearing its song. That's because every experience we have ever had of a bird prior to that moment is now involved in our experience. This means that reactivity and (mis-)interpretation play out a lot in our relationships. Here are some examples. For one, acronyms have become commonplace, especially when texting, and, as we have perhaps all discovered, provide lots of room for misinterpretation. LOL can be laugh out loud or lots of love, TGIF can be thank goodness it's Friday or This grandma is fabulous. Emojis are much the same. 😊 can mean many things—a joke, irony, flirtation, or maybe just positive vibes. At work, my team has often had colleagues for whom English is their second language. We have developed a humorous list of translations to avoid misunderstandings. Here are a few examples:

What the English say	What the English mean	What anyone else understands
Very interesting	I don't agree/that's a terrible idea.	They are impressed.
I'll bear it in mind.	I will do nothing about it.	They will probably do it.
This is in no sense a rebuke.	I am furious with you and letting you know it.	I am not cross with you.
QUITE good (with the stress on the "quite")	A bit disappointing	Quite good
Quite GOOD (with the stress on the "good")	Excellent	Quite good

So, our reactions are consequences of how we interpret a situation, not necessarily the facts of the situation. And, acronyms, emojis, and words can be interpreted in different ways. Very often we are not aware of the interpretation; we're just left with our reactions.

The Barefoot Professor: Gazelles and Humans

Gazelles living in a savannah work as a social group. Together they move to where there is grazing or water, or shelter. They work together, always keeping watch for danger. When all is well, their minds and bodies remain alert but register safety, togetherness, and they can get on with grazing. If on the other hand a gazelle senses change or danger, maybe a cheetah, it alerts the group, they all orient to the danger, and get ready to act. This might gather into a tight group for protection, perhaps with the young in the middle of the group. Or they may run from danger. They may outrun the cheetah, or possibly an old or sick gazelle falls prey to it. But here is the thing. As soon as the danger passes, the gazelle's minds and bodies settle back down to normality and return to grazing. We have a lot in common with gazelles in terms of the structure and function of our brains and bodies, and much of the sensing, alerting, and call to action gazelles have is pretty well the same in human minds and bodies. **But here is the key difference.** We can *re-create* the past in imagination and *create possible futures* in this moment. Imagine a gazelle prone to anxiety, after the danger had passed. You'd see a thought bubble over its head in which there is always a cheetah—this is a gazelle with generalized anxiety. Or maybe the thought bubble has in it the old gazelle that fell prey to the cheetah, with a narrative "Poor Hank, why him? He didn't deserve that; I bet it will be me next." This is the gazelle prone to depression. This is of course what we humans sometimes do—we overthink.

Getting to Know How Sensations, Emotions, Actions, and Thoughts Write Our Script

To recognize and move past feeling overwhelmed, anxious, exhausted, to recapture our mojo, it helps to unpack what is going on. The best way to do this is to take the time to become familiar with how your body sensations, emotions, impulses, and thoughts work together. Think of what's going on as a four-part model:

1. **Bodily sensations**. In any moment your body is a myriad of transitory sensations: tightness, ease, contraction, temperature, pressure, tingling, pulsing, and so on. Through practices like the Body Scan you become much more familiar with body sensations.

2. **Emotions**. Classically, psychologists have categorized some emotions as basic or elementary (happiness, anger, surprise, sadness, disgust, fear). Others are seen as more complex, perhaps combining several emotions (humility is a combination of self-awareness and freedom from pride). Others involve

thinking; they add a story (gratitude, "I am so glad that happened," or disappointment, "I am so upset that happened"). They can be on a scale—you can be contented, happy, really happy, or ecstatic. They have a hedonic tone, meaning simply they can be experienced as pleasant or unpleasant. Finally, you have a sense of emotions in your body, each having its own signature.

3. **Impulses and actions.** Impulses (or urges) are like calls to action; our body–mind is inclined to act in a particular way. This can be either quite basic (fight, flee, or freeze) or more developed (step back and take stock). We can also think of impulses on a scale. For example, at any time, your state of arousal can be quite sluggish or tired (+1 or 2 on a 10-point scale) up to being really activated and energized (6–10, on a 10-point scale). Emotions are often associated with a call to action, happiness is often expansive, anger can lead us to strike out, fear can lead us to fight, flee, or freeze. More complex emotions can have correspondingly more complex impulses associated with them. For example, humility can help us recognize when we have done something good or well and moderates our response. In contrast pride can motivate us to act big-headed; hence the saying, "pride before the fall."

4. **Thoughts, images, remembering, planning, daydreaming, thinking in all its forms**. The thinking realm is extraordinary, so rich and interesting. We can imagine the future, reconstruct the past, plan, imagine whole worlds. We tell ourselves stories; we like to have stories with a beginning, a middle and an end, with a good guy and a bad guy. As I said in Chapter 3, thinking can be our friend or it can work against us.

This simple way of describing the landscape of our body and mind enables us to answer these questions: "What is happening for me right now?" "What's going on in my body?" "What moods or emotions are around?" "What impulses are around?" "What am I thinking?" "Are there any images?"

Unpacking our experience into these four parts is the first step—it separates out and illuminates what's happening. A soupy mess, like feeling overwhelmed, becomes clearer, separated out and more detailed. It highlights the connections between our thoughts and feelings, how bodily states shape our impulses and so on.

At first you may have trouble distinguishing bodily sensations from emotions and from thoughts. Is anxiety a body sensation or an emotion? Is embarrassment a feeling or a thought? Try to see it as a process of discovery, bringing a lightness of touch and curiosity to your experience. Anxiety is typically made up of all four parts of the model, and seeing this can be an important part of the process of working with the sensations, impulses, and thoughts. Our immediate interpretations are typically quick and automatic. It takes time and practice to be able to step back and see them happening. You may well find you're doing a reconstruction after the fact. That's okay, because it's part of the learning to step back and take a different perspective. It may be that you can't do much about your first reaction, but you might be able to catch the layers of further reactivity we sometimes pile on. Greater awareness of the (often so rapid) way in which our interpretation shapes and is shaped by what is happening in our bodies and minds can bring freedom and choice.

Using Our Natural Resources in Real Life, for Life

A good place to start learning to see the four parts of the model in action is with the good things that happen in your day-to-day life. Every day, even full busy days will have moments that are enjoyable, amusing, playful, remarkable, revitalizing, even laugh-out-loud—if you bring curiosity and open-mindedness to your day.

Exploring Pleasant Events

Think back to what you discovered in the appreciation practice in Chapter 4.
Here are some examples:

- Being symptom free the first day after a heavy cold. Appreciating the sense of physical health, vitality, and clarity of thought—and being able to breathe
- A funny meme that that makes you laugh out loud
- The greeting of a pet
- After a busy day, the moment of "putting your feet up"

The Barefoot Professor: Awareness of Pleasant Experiences

Research shows that awareness of pleasant experiences—small momentary things—and enjoying them as they contribute to overall mental health and well-being. Studies have shown that psychological approaches that teach how to develop awareness of pleasant experiences work well because they help people develop their "positive valence system"—the ability to recognize and enjoy the positive in our lives. One reason mindfulness training is effective is that it helps people learn this skill. Contentment and happiness are learnable skills.

The Experiences Calendar is a tool to help you notice and unpack moments throughout your day. If it feels helpful, use it to notice and write down one pleasant experience each day. But this is not supposed to be hard work. It's helping you do what you're already doing, but in a new way. If the calendar doesn't feel useful, do it in whatever way helps this become a part of your life, recognizing and savoring good experiences.

Instead of freewheeling through pleasant moments, try intentionally paying attention to the sensing, feeling, and thinking elements of the experience. What do you discover when you become more aware of the elements of your experience?

EXERCISE: **Experiences Calendar**

You can download one from the Mindfulness for Life website.

What was the experience?	Sensations	Emotions	Behaviors	Thoughts
	What did your body feel, in detail, during this experience?	What moods and feelings accompanied the experience?	What impulses or behaviors did you notice?	What thoughts or images went through your mind?

Here is Ling's calendar entry from watching TV one evening.

What was the experience?	Sensations	Emotions	Behaviors	Thoughts
	What did your body feel, in detail, during this experience?	What moods and feelings accompanied the experience?	What impulses or behaviors did you notice?	What thoughts or images went through your mind?
Watching a funny show on TV one evening	Comfortable, warm, supported by the sofa, stroking the cat	Fun, relaxed	Laughter	These characters are so relatable and likable.

LING: *I tried this when I was watching TV one evening, but then I ended up feeling bad. I had all these thoughts: "You are way too busy for this." "You haven't earned this." "You're a single mother; you have so much to do—stop being a princess."*

After a full day watching TV, stroking the cat was a good moment for Ling. But it also reveals how Ling's negative thinking can contaminate good moments. Knowing this, she could nip it in the bud by having a little word with herself: "*Whoa, that's harsh, Ling. I absolutely need to take care of myself, precisely because I am busy and a mum.*"

This deceptively simple four-part model can be used to describe pretty well any moment, pleasant moments (like Ling watching a funny show on TV), upsetting moments (like Ling's friend not waving back), or moments that we normally regard as filler moments as we move through our day (waiting for a bus or train). Practice with moments that enrich your day and see what it is like to pause and unpack, even savor these moments. Normally, it's easiest to practice this with pleasant experiences and then work up to unpleasant experiences (which you'll do in the next chapter).

Understanding our senses and unpacking our experience isn't a navel-gazing exercise—it's intended for use in real life. It's also not supposed to be a one-off Band-Aid. It's for life. Let's turn to an aspect of real life we are all familiar with: our smartphones. How much time do you spend on your phone? Is it more or less than you would like? How much of this time is intentional?

In this practice you explore how you relate to your phone or to digital devices more broadly. Try to have as open a mind as you can as you do this—so much of what we do on our phones is habitual. See if you can come at this with interest, patience, nonjudgment—adopt beginner's mind to step out of habit.

PRACTICE: **Mindfulness of Your Digital Device**

You can follow along on our website.

Before starting, switch off your phone and put it down in front of you. Take a few moments to stabilize and anchor your attention. When you're ready, do each of the following, noticing after each action what is happening to the four elements of your experience—sensations, emotions, impulses or actions, thoughts or imagery:

1. Take your phone and hold it in your hand, without switching it on.
2. Switch the phone on and just register its turning on, the home screen opening up.

3. Now open the app or function that you use most often, possibly even overuse. Register what comes up in this app, but don't interact with it just yet.
4. Go ahead and interact with the app, doing what you normally do.

So, what did you notice? What did you learn at each step of this exercise in terms of body sensations, feelings, impulses, and thoughts?

LING: *I sometimes say to my kids, "Get off your phones; it will rot your brain." And they respond, "But Mum, you spend as much time on your phone as we do, and sometimes I have to say, 'Mum' three times to get your attention because you're so caught up in your phone." I know they're right; I do spend a lot of time on my phone, and sometimes I scroll for hours through Instagram.*

So, what did I notice in this practice? Well, I realized that I kind of felt a heady mixture of anxiety and excitement as I picked up the phone. My finger was literally trembling a little bit as I held back from starting to open Instagram. Then I scrolled through some of the people I follow, including my kids, to find out what they're up to! Once I opened the app I kind of lost touch with myself; it was like water disappearing down the drain. Now I feel a bit shell shocked. Too much awareness isn't necessarily a good thing! (laughing)

Most people spend quite a bit of time on digital devices, many feeling they spend too much time. There is a lot to learn from bringing awareness to how you interact with your phone using the four-part model. Consider the moment you reach for your phone (behavior), perhaps in a moment of boredom (emotion), with the thought "I wonder if anything interesting has happened since I last looked at my phone." When you start to recognize and separate out the feelings and thoughts, and the associated underlying sensations (maybe restlessness or agitation), you have a chance to notice the impulse to reach for your phone and what's driving it— maybe to escape the feelings of boredom and restlessness. Explore when you tend to pick up your phone during your day. Ask, "Why am I picking up my phone? What else could I do to recognize and respond to what I'm feeling and thinking right now?" If you're bored, can you get interested in the boredom (instead of trying to escape it) and ask, "Can I be okay with this, doing nothing?" "Or my impulse is to check Instagram—insert your own top distraction on your phone—can I at least do it with some awareness and see what that's like?" This can be unsettling. But any genuine learning can be unsettling because you're opening to something new. Here is a radical idea: maybe boredom is interesting.

> Maybe boredom is like a veil, and looking behind it reveals something worth paying attention to.

*The Barefoot Professor: Are Smartphones Weapons
of Mass Distraction?*

We've been programmed to use our phones in ways that make us feel better in
the short term—this type of learning (associative learning and negative reinforcement) is very powerful; it has a compulsive quality to it. This is no accident. The people who design phones and the apps have extensive knowledge
and expertise in the psychology of attention, motivation, behavior, behavior
change, and addiction. They have used psychology to first grab your attention,
then keep your attention and drive you to places that may interest you. But I
am sorry to say, they are not working for you. They are working for the companies that produce the apps, serving their clients, investors, and shareholders.
This means their agenda is normally to sell you something (trainers, gaming
apps, golf equipment, knitting patterns). They want you to engage as much
as possible and to build who you are following and your followers, so they can
do more of the same. This isn't a conspiracy theory. It's business; the apps are
designed to create revenue, using different business models, but all premised
on capturing and keeping your attention. It's not my opinion; it's what many
of the people who have worked in this industry have said. Many of them don't
allow their own kids to use the very technology they developed.

Why introduce mindfulness of your smartphone at this stage? Because
mindfulness can be used in every area of your life. Once some basic mindfulness skills are in place, you can use them everywhere and anytime. So, what you
learn when you bring awareness to our digital devices can be incredibly free-
ing. It moves us from being captivated by our digital devices to choosing how
we use our phones, so they serve us rather than enslave us. How about spring
cleaning your phone? Which apps bring you joy, connect you with people you
love, and otherwise serve you? Put those on the homepage. Which waste your
time, are used as escapism, or make you feel worse? Can you delete them, at
least for a while, or put them on another screen, out of sight? Can you change
how you relate to your phone? Can you put it away from you when you're sleeping, have a break from it for an hour or more before you go to bed? Where are
the chargers? Would it help to move them somewhere that gives you a chance
to consider if and how to use your phone? How about having a trial separation
from your phone, in the way couples sometimes do, to reevaluate their relationship? It could be an hour, a day, a week. This can be helpful in answering
some important questions: what apps are essential, maybe the ones you use to
communicate with loved ones and maps; which you enjoy as a guilty pleasure;
and which you didn't miss at all, in fact, feeling better without them? Each time
you notice the pull to your device, ask, "Is this serving me? What might serve
me better in this moment?" When you use it, can you keep your awareness, so

you have a sense of how what you're doing is affecting your body and mind? At the end of your trial separation, like couples who do this, you may discover you love your phone or that your life is better without it. Or perhaps it's a good relationship but you need to work on it.

Getting to Know How Sensations, Emotions, Actions, and Thoughts Shape and Are Shaped by Our Lives

Someone not returning our greeting, a date where there is chemistry, a friend's kindness. . . . All these moments shape our day, and over time our lives. What I'd like to do next is add a fifth part to the model. How is it possible that we react to the same situation differently at different times?

Imagine you're in a lousy mood, all your plans for your day have fallen through, and you text a good friend in the morning: "Hi, what's up? Would you like to meet up?" You can see your friend has read the message, but there is no response all day long. Now imagine you're in a good mood, you have a full day planned, and you text the same message to the same friend. Again, you see they've read the message and don't respond. You're in a good mood and you get on with the rest of your day. In these two scenarios, how do you react? What's happening in your body, what do you feel, what do you do, what do you think? Typically, our prevailing state of body–mind "shapes" and "flavors" our interpretations. If we're in a bad mood, we see things more negatively. If we're in a good mood, we see things more positively. And that plays out over time. Our interpretations can make a bad mood hang around and even get worse. Or they can help us shake something off and move on. This scenario will likely play out differently on a day that is empty or full simply because we have more or less time to worry and ruminate. Context is the fifth part of the model, the way our state of body–mind shapes and is shaped by our lives.

Who or What Is Shaping Our Minds and Bodies?

We like and crave pleasure. We look for what makes us feel good—sweet food, stimulation from gaming, web surfing, drinking, shopping, scrolling on our phones, hedonistic pleasures. On one level this may seem innocent and benign. But it can have a downside. The first is that the good feeling is momentary and, more often than not, when we get what we want, it is simply followed by the next thing we want. This craving drives our mind to turn momentary experiences into dissatisfaction because we have this sense of a gap between how things are and how they should be. In our evolutionary story these drives helped us find water, food, safety, and so on, but in the modern world they can be less helpful. Why? Because our desires are rarely satisfied, and our attempts tend to just strengthen them.

> ### The Ancient Oak: "Unquenchable Thirst"
>
> There is an ancient Pali word, *tanha,* that the Buddha used to describe what he discovered about craving as he carefully studied his own mind. It is sometimes translated as craving for stimulation, for a sense of being and feeling okay. It also means trying to get away from feeling uncomfortable, or bad or anything negative. It's sometimes translated as desire. But the best way to understand it is *like a thirst that can't be satisfied by drinking.* However much you drink, the thirst remains. You hear about people who were stranded at sea, surrounded by saltwater, knowing that drinking the saltwater cannot stop their thirst.

> SAM: *I LOVE sneakers. I worked really hard to afford these Jordans. When I put them on the first time, my whole vibe changed—my "swagger" hit a new level. But here's the thing, the hype only lasted a minute before my phone started bombarding me with the next must-have sneakers. Retro Jordans? Yup, needed those too. It's a never-ending cycle. My room looks like a shoe warehouse, and I'm constantly hustling to sell the ones I don't need anymore.*

This craving can come from a sense of discomfort and not being able to tolerate it. We're trying to escape bad feelings, even ourselves, by making ourselves feel good—anything different from how we feel. This reinforces craving, because the hit we get from shopping, gaming, scrolling through our phones, and so on makes us feel better for a minute.

Wanting and craving can take on more elaborate forms as we strive to be the person we think we ought to be, to have the sort of life we think we're supposed to have. There are so many messages about being admired, successful,

> Mindfulness involves leaving the waiting room for a better future, to be fully present in this moment. How can you step out of this waiting room?

and loved. We see people around us having lives we think are better than ours—their house is better, their kids better adjusted, their vacations better, their lives in more control. We want to be like them, strive to match them. Advertisers and social media companies are experts in this branch of psychology. They know how to grab our attention, exploit this craving, and sell us things that will help us feel better. This striving to be someone other than who we are sabotages our well-being, our health, our ability to live meaningful lives. They have succeeded in making us feel like we are not good enough, that we are lacking something in ourselves and in our lives. This takes us away from this moment and into a future in which we imagine having the things that will make us happy. This moment becomes a waiting room for a better future. Understandably, the perfect person, perfect life we yearn for remains elusive. Not surprisingly, this rather unpleasant waiting room is one we want to escape.

As I already mentioned at the start of this chapter, what you're learning are the (deceptively) simple foundation stones for building the life you imagine. When you use these ideas to make sense of your experience over time, you start to see things you couldn't see before, in more detail; you can see how the landscape of your body–mind unfolds and changes.

For example, fatigue is an interesting state of body–mind that compromises well-being. It's variously described as "feeling wiped out," "limbs feeling heavy as lead," "bones like glass, fragile and brittle," "mind like fog," "weariness like a heavy cloak." It's a common experience and can point to all sorts of causes—sleep deprivation obviously, but also chronic stress, diet, dehydration, hormonal changes, extreme heat or cold, medications, and illness. Recognizing fatigue is vitally important because it helps us potentially redress its causes.

Putting Our Body–Mind to Work in Our Lives

The moment at which you classify your experience as pleasant, unpleasant, or neutral is the key. As you start to recognize and separate out your sensations, moods, impulses, and thoughts, a subtle and important insight is available. You can notice the moment at which experiences are *categorized as pleasant, unpleasant, or neutral.* This very early link in the chain is important because it dictates how your experience unfolds. Categorizing an experience as unpleasant typically triggers some attempt to fix it (problem solving, worry, or rumination) or avoidance. We're going to explore that in the next chapter. Categorizing a moment as pleasant typically triggers wanting more—craving. Pleasure is not in and of itself bad. There's nothing wrong with Sam's liking sneakers and enjoying his "swagger." It's when it becomes compulsive, when wanting is never satisfied, when we think we're not good enough because we don't have something—this all creates a sense of dissatisfaction.

How can you savor all that is good in a way that supports a good life? By bringing awareness to this moment of categorizing your experience, you can start to shape how it unfolds. You can unpack these experiences, and this supports your capacity for appreciation, joy, care, and contentment. It is a chance to turn a pleasant fragment of experience into appreciation or meet an unpleasant fragment with friendliness and care.

PRACTICE: **Savoring Good Moments**

You can follow along on our website.

Bring to mind a time from today or the last few days when you felt good, had a sense of fun, meaning, connection, happiness. Once you've settled on something, bring the memory into focus. Maybe run it like a video in your mind's eye from beginning to end. As you do this:

What's happening in your body? What sensations do you experience, where, how intensely, maybe your face, chest, torso. . . . ?

What moods or emotions are around? Lightly notice and maybe name them.

What do you feel like doing? This may be something personal to you, like really taking the time to enjoy the moment or maybe doing something, like reaching out to someone, sending a text maybe.

What thoughts and images are around?

What did you notice? It can be interesting to explore how these moments unfold, the links in the chain I referred to above. At what moment does the mind decide this is pleasant? What happens next? Seeing and understanding these links in the chain is the basis for both breaking the links that create distress and strengthening links that support your well-being.

There is so much to appreciate in the world. Sam's list included sneakers, for sure. Sophia's list included taking in waves breaking on a beach, cooking for friends, live music, laughing with her daughter, and tart crisp apples. My list includes the first coffee of the day, swimming, and spending time with people I love.

> What's on your list of things to appreciate in the world? How has it changed over the years?

Standing Up to Our Inner Judge

I remember being with a friend having a cup of tea in a café overlooking the coastline and saying: "This is so beautiful. I wish I lived on the coast." He replied, without any agenda, "Yes, and isn't it also good to just enjoy this moment?" This took me aback because I realized he was right. I smiled and came back to enjoying my friend's company, our tea in the café, and the amazing view.

As this example illustrates, after labeling something as pleasant or unpleasant, the next link in the chain is our inner judge, passing sentence. Is it good, bad, or indifferent, worthy or unworthy, needs attention or can be ignored? This is what I did at the café with my friend. Rather than simply appreciate this moment an inner judge had said, "I don't live somewhere as nice as this. I wish I did." I had turned a good experience into a judgment about my life.

The judge is also a bit of a problem solver; everything needs solving, even things that don't. With unpleasant moments, the judge says, "I don't like this. How can I get rid of it or fix it?" More than this, our inner judge likes to over-think things, ruminate about the past, worry about the future, and compare ourselves with others, both downward ("I am better than") or upward ("I am worse than"). In both cases, we've lost contact with the direct experience in the moment. Mindfulness helps us first see the judge and know when it is unhelpful and when it is helpful. When it's unhelpful, diminishing my moment in a café with a friend, we can stand up to it, and when it's helpful, we can follow its advice.

Creating a New Habit
of Paying Attention to Our Body–Mind

Get into the habit of stopping when you notice something happening in your body–mind—a bodily sensation, emotion, impulse, or a thought—and asking "What is this? What is this telling me or pointing to?" Our body–mind, like a smartphone battery, has a readout of its energy level—"fully charged," or "good to go, charged, green light," or "need recharging," or "critical." Notice when your body is rested and energized and how powerfully this shapes whether something unexpected is interpreted as exciting or scary. This in turn shapes an impulse to either act or hide away. If you feel well rested, you're better able to handle what the day throws at you. In contrast, if you're tired, everything in your day can become difficult, too hard, and you're more likely to give yourself a hard time. So sleep and rest are important, and if you're tired, you need to take special care about what you do and say and look after yourself. When we're young, we're unaware of how tired we may be, and we keep going. That's why babies scream with crankiness—they don't know what's making them feel so bad or what to do about it. When we're older, we might recognize that the second half of our day goes way better if we take a 20-minute power nap.

Emotions can signal what is happening and what is needed in any given moment. For example, shame suggests something has made us feel less than, not okay. Sometimes that someone is us! The shame may be misplaced (our tendency to be our own worst critics), but sometimes it isn't (we've done something that violates our values, and shame here helps us put it right). Our energy level, our emotions—these are just examples of the whole body–mind landscape. Seeing how the five parts of this model—context, body sensations, emotions, impulses, and thoughts—interact is a fascinating and endless study. You can explore every element of the model and how they all fit together for a lifetime.

Paying Attention to the Moments That Matter

You've started to explore what matters most, your values, and what you appreciate in your life. Paying particular attention to these moments clarifies and strengthens our values and aligns our lives with our values. For most people, family and friends are really important and the source of great joy and sometimes also real difficulties. Yet we all fall into the habit of listening to people with only half an ear. In a group it can be as if people are in a stack, just waiting for their turn to speak, rehearsing the story or point they want to talk about, even as others are speaking. In the following practice, the 50–50 practice introduced on page 65, you can use mindfulness to help you listen and speak mindfully.

PRACTICE: Deep Listening and Speaking

Choose someone you care about, someone you really value. Next time you are with them, as they speak, try listening like your life depended on it, really giving them airtime. As you do this, what do you notice in your body–mind? When it is your turn to speak, pause, just for a second or two, and see if you can stay aware of what is happening in your body–mind as you start to speak and then as you are speaking.

SAM: *So, I'm out on this date, and I knew early on I like this guy, I'm going to want to see him again. Then this thought creeps in: "What if he's not feeling it and doesn't want to see me again?" Instant anxiety.*

So I pull this move. I ask him two questions that are super interesting: "What animal would you have as a pet?" and "Why?" He said, "A donkey," and I crack up. Then he explains it's because of all their traits, loyalty, loving, a bit cantankerous. While he's talking, I listen with my full attention—well, almost. I track that I'm interested, feet safe, still anxiety, but much less, amused, and, boom, chemistry! And he's picking up on that—he has my full attention and he's feeling the chemistry too—I can see him relax. He starts talking even more freely. And I know it's pop psychology, but I explained the question is also about the kind of person and relationship a person is looking for. We properly belly-laughed.

Staying Safe

In Chapter 2 I introduced the idea that our attention naturally functions as our built-in protector—a bit like the gatekeeper of a walled city, the bouncer in a nightclub, or the antivirus software on our computer, flagging threats, knowing what is toxic, and protecting us. All the ideas in this chapter can be used to help you stay safe. For example, in deep listening, our body–mind will tell us who is safe and who we need to be wary of, when words are well-intentioned or not. We can see the impulse to move toward something because it is safe or away from it because it is threatening. When we need to rest and recharge. We can see which thoughts are easy and natural and which are uncomfortable and that we try to keep out. Or if they found their way in, we try to eject them.

SOPHIA: *Being, even feeling, criticized is really triggering for me. I freeze and lock down.*

MOHAMMED: *When my back pain becomes intense, and persists, the thought "This is unbearable" is terrifying. I feel helpless and hopeless, and I seize up, and that makes the pain worse. Honestly, I think, "I can't live with this."*

Sophia and Mohammed are describing the different elements of their experience, how they feed each other. You have to pay attention, or at least leave the space for protective mindfulness—without recognizing these moments, the mind's protective tendencies can't step in. But it can also help you learn that sometimes what you thought was dangerous is safe and vice versa. There are skills you're learning as you go along.

Finally, we are all different. Some of us are very tuned in to our bodies, or aspects of our bodies, but not our thoughts. Some of us live in our heads and have no idea what's happening in our body, until it grabs our attention because it is in pain, sick, going through puberty, menopause, and so on. There is also evidence that even though we may think we're tuned in to our bodies, we're not as accurate as we think we are.

SAM: *OMG, puberty. Total nightmare. Felt like I was the last one of everyone I knew to hit puberty. I acted like I didn't give a damn, including to myself. I pulled on this geekiness cloak, acting like I was a tech and gaming wizard. I guess it was a safety cloak—my way of staying safe. But recently I've been turning to paying attention to my body and seeing what helps: at work, to feel more confident, with self-talk like "You've got this, Sam," to have that sense of "hell yes." I guess feeling comfortable in my own skin, and in my love life being able to be myself, give and take and let go. (Smiling) I'm not nerdy. I'm a ninja.*

LING: *A few months ago I was having some mood swings, not like anything I was used to, and had this kind of brain fog, I'd wake in the middle of the night wide awake. But I just got on with my life. It was only when my periods started becoming irregular that I thought, "What's happening?" I made an appointment with my doctor, and she said I was going into perimenopause and offered me hormone replacement patches. Duh, how did I not know that? How did I miss what my body was telling me? I've really noticed how the patches have helped my thinking, sleep, and mood.*

Having a Sense of Control Over Life Means Using Our Natural Resources to the Fullest

Our experience is a continual stream of sensing, feeling, and thinking. Our minds are very good at summarizing; at giving us the metadata, predicting what is about to happen, and if any action is needed. Becoming more familiar with the landscape of body–mind means going beyond the metadata, going back to the richness of our direct experience unfolding moment by moment. This can be very normalizing (all minds and bodies do this) and can be a great teacher (when I am tired, I am prone to think negatively and act impulsively). The five-part model and Experiences Calendar can support you to begin to describe the elements of your experience, and in doing so, you begin to see how experience is created and what happens next. It's a lifelong journey to develop this familiarity, sensitivity, and intimacy with your mind and body. Foundation stones aren't visible, but they are so important to everything you'll build in the chapters ahead. If at any time you want to strengthen the foundations, even if it isn't the most exciting thing to do, revisit this chapter and the work of familiarizing yourself with your body–mind.

6

How We React to Stress and Difficulties

Between stimulus and reactivity, there is no space,
No awareness, no chance to check your compass or map.

When something difficult happens, how do you tend to react? Think back to the last few times you felt stressed. What did you do? Was there something that you kind of knew wasn't a good idea, was maybe a bit "reactive," but it made you feel a little better? Sometimes it's easier to spot reactivity in our best friends and close family. If you don't know, ask someone who knows you well if they'll answer this question for you, kindly and honestly.

SAM: *When I'm feeling like I need an escape, I've got this go-to move—grab my phone. It's like I can vanish into that thing for hours. Or, you know, I'll dive into some gaming. It's like being an ostrich with its head in the sand. It's my way of dodging boredom, shaking off the tired vibes, or, especially in the evenings, ditching all the leftover work baggage from the day. It's my getaway.*

LING: *I've been prone to feeling low since I was a teenager. I get this knot in my stomach, a real sense of dread. It's as if Niagara Falls is just around the next bend in the river and I am being sucked toward it—out of control and scary—not a good feeling at all. So, to make myself feel better I do one of two things—paddle harder (get busy) or pretend it isn't happening. Of course, I know, deep down, this won't work, but I feel that at least I'm doing something; and that sort of helps.*

MOHAMMED: *I go into my own shell. It is not as if I am doing it deliberately; it just happens. My wife will try and try to get a reaction out of me, and I just go farther into my shell. And the next thing I know everyone is grumpy and you could cut the atmosphere with a knife. But, and I don't like admitting this, somehow inside my shell I feel safe. I am not proud, but it's what I do.*

SOPHIA: *My daughter said to me, "Mum, you can't eat your feelings." I had to laugh. I see myself walking into the kitchen to the cupboard with the snack food. I know, sort of, I said to myself I wouldn't, but I do it anyway. Then I don't like myself for doing it, even feel disgusted with myself sometimes when it goes too far, and I eat like a whole pack of cookies.*

These are examples of typical things that we all do to avoid feeling bad. In this chapter you're going to explore your habitual ways of reacting, particularly when they don't serve you well in your life. To do this you need first to steady your attention and become more aware of what is happening, which you learned to do in Chapters 2 and 3. Then, you need to unpack experiences by breaking them down into sensations, feelings, urges, and thoughts, which you learned in Chapter 5. These foundational skills are what will enable you to start to see your reactivity more clearly in this chapter. This can feel a bit like focusing on all that is wrong, which can easily feel a bit discouraging. But if you're to have a chance to respond in ways more aligned with your values, the life you imagined, you need first to see and understand reactivity.

Learning to Recognize Our Patterns of Reactivity

We touch something hot, and we instinctively pull back our hand. We are primed to react in these ways. Someone we love is sad, and we reach out to comfort them. We see a beautiful sunset or rainbow, and we have a sense of wonder.

How can we make sense of this? As you've already discovered, we label everything as pleasant, unpleasant, or just neutral, often even without being aware of it. If it's labeled unpleasant or pleasant, it may trigger a reaction. So we pull back our hand from a hot plate; we reach out to someone who is sad. We also tend to judge everything and then tell ourselves stories about what is happening. "I am such an idiot for touching the hot pan." "I hope I haven't upset my friend." "I wish I lived somewhere where I could sit on the porch and see a sunset like this every day, but I can't afford to." These stories are often about how we think things should be, how we'd like them to be, how things have been in the past, or how we think they might be in the future. This can turn an unpleasant or even a pleasant moment into something else altogether.

Why Do We Do Things That Don't Help Us in the Long Term?

More than 2,500 years ago, the Buddha told the story of the two arrows to describe how we turn pain into suffering. We all encounter pain and discomfort, which is the first arrow, an automatic, simple reaction to something like touching a live flame or being stung by a bee. But then there's a second arrow—this is our resistance, judgments, and the stories we tell ourselves. The first arrow, the pain of being burnt by the flame, is automatic. It will be fired regardless, and there is nothing we can do about it. The second arrow is how we react, and it is here that we, largely without knowing we're doing it, can create distress and suffering.

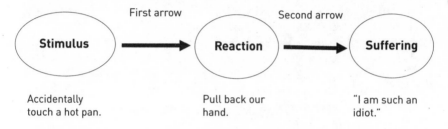

The Barefoot Professor: Why We Do Things That Don't Help Us

Evolutionary and behavioral psychology has expanded the Buddha's idea of the two arrows. The tendency to react automatically to things that happen in our external world is hardwired. In our evolutionary history it helped us meet our basic needs for safety, water, food, shelter, companionship. In our personal histories too, we've learned strategies that have worked for us. They made us feel safe, helped us feel better. A child growing up in a home where there was a lot of conflict may become very adept at avoidance, just like an ostrich sticking its head in the sand. He may learn to avoid the upsetting conflict by withdrawing to his room and putting on some headphones with music.

Behavioral psychology describes powerful conditions for learning. First, *associative learning* simply means that we learn which stimuli create which responses. My dog learned to associate my taking off my shoes with staying home, so he'd quickly settle. Putting on my shoes meant a walk might be in the cards. In mindfulness practice we can start to see how thoughts, emotions, impulses, and bodily states are associated with one another. *Operant learning* takes this to the next level; this is where something we do has an effect. My dog would do anything for a food treat, so I could teach him to sit, come when I called him, lie down, walk to heel all by simply giving him a treat when he did what I wanted. We're no different; we've learned to respond to praise, work harder for bonuses, show loyalty to stores because we get loyalty points. These are all examples of operant learning through *positive reinforcement*.

An important version of this is *negative reinforcement*. This simply means something we do has the effect of making a bad feeling go away. We don't like our children whining, so we may give in to them to make the whining go away. This inadvertently reinforces the whining. Powerful contemporary examples are painkillers, which we can become physically and psychologically addicted to because they numb pain. One theory of self-injury is that it is reinforcing because it numbs pain. Punishment works in a similar way; we don't do things because we learn that when we do something bad will happen. Where I live there are speed cameras on the roads, and no one speeds because there is a very high chance of getting a speeding ticket.

Associative learning is very powerful, and behaviors fade slowly even if the associations are no longer there. My dog carried on coming when I called him, even if I had no snacks. But even more important to know is that the best way to keep a behavior alive is to reinforce it only some of the time (called *partial* or *intermittent reinforcement*). Why do we carry on doing things long after they serve us? This is simply because they either haven't faded (psychologists call this *extinction*) or more likely they're reinforced sometimes.

So why do we react in ways that are ultimately unhelpful? Why do we fire a second arrow? In some ways the answer is obvious. We don't want to feel bad; we don't like it. We want to feel good. We want things to go well, and we want them to continue going well. Busyness, sticking our head in the sand, blaming someone else, trying desperately to "fix it"—these strategies often make us feel like we're doing something helpful, trying to fix or explain what's happened. They may even make us feel better some of the time. Because we feel a little bit better, we may do it again and again, and before we know it has become a habit, even part of our personality.

> Reactivity is a completely understandable but misguided attempt to help us feel a bit better.

Of course, many difficult things we face in our lives are only too real (illness, money problems, losing people we love, as well as wider issues in the world like inequalities, economic downturns, climate change). But with these issues, how we react, the second arrow, determines how much distress and suffering we will experience. The hopeful message is that you can come to recognize our reactivity, the second arrow, and in time realize that firing the second arrow is optional.

> Because reactivity is so automatic, we may not realize that we don't have to fire the second arrow.

SAM: *I can't stand my psoriasis. It's haunted me since I was a kid, and when I have an outbreak, it's like a full-on attack of second arrows. It's not fair. I scratch even though I know it's gonna make it worse, and I get into beating myself up.*

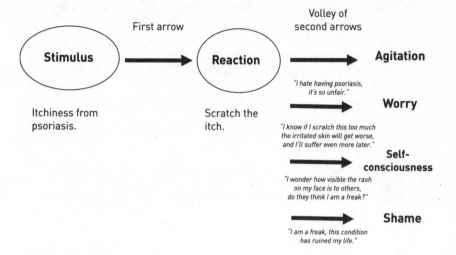

PRACTICE: **Recognizing Reactivity Using the Vicious Flower**

How can you recognize your patterns of reactivity? The best way to understand your mind's reactivity is to use what you've already learned to stabilize and gather your attention and then watch what's happening in your body and mind when you're stressed. Psychologists developed a tool called the *vicious flower* to help us do this. It shows how in moments of stress we can go down well-worn paths of unhelpful behaviors and thoughts:

Step 1. *Start by anchoring yourself in your breath and body.* If you're going to look at your reactivity, it helps to feel present and steady as a first step.

Step 2. *Bring to mind some emotional or relationship problem that has happened to you recently—the sort of problem that tends to tangle you up, where you get a sense of "Ah, yes, I've been here before. This is what happens to me."* It might be the sort of situation that creates feelings of guilt, shame, sadness, anger, resentment, or irritability. Choose something manageable, that you can work with, not something overwhelming. Trust your protective mindfulness to know what feels right and doable in this moment. If it simply doesn't feel right, trust that and step away from the exercise.

Once you've chosen something, recall a specific recent example. Sharpen the image or play through the memory of what happened like a video in your mind. Really tune in to the experience, as if it were happening right now.

Step 3. *Unpack it*, using the four-part model. Note what's happening in this situation in your body (any sensations), your mood, any impulses or calls to action, thoughts, or images. You're taking what happened for you and separating it out so you can stand back and see the landscape of your body and mind more clearly. Keep it simple—a word or phrase to describe the different parts of your experience.

Step 4. *Now ask yourself these questions:*

What did you find yourself doing and thinking?

How did you try to make yourself feel better? What else, including things you kind of knew were probably unhelpful?

What happens when you do these things? How does it play out?

Step 5. *Use the vicious flower to capture your ways of coping with pain and distress.*

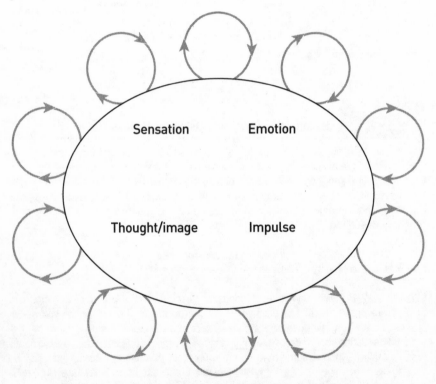

Sensation   Emotion

Thought/image   Impulse

**The Vicious Flower: How distress and suffering can be maintained
and even made worse.**

The middle oval is what was happening in your body and mind in the moment reactivity is kindled. Start by writing in the circle any sensations, emotions, impulses, and thoughts. Just a word or two will normally do; no need to get it perfect or to write an essay.

Next, take all the ways you thought of to try to fix the problem. These are more than likely all very human and understandable ways of trying to cope, to help you feel better. For each strategy you came up with, ask yourself, "What happens when I do this?" And here is the key question: Does this coping strategy support your well-being over time, overall, in different situations? Is it a choice or more a habit? Is it helpful or in the scheme of things unhelpful, maybe even destructive? If it doesn't help overall, it makes things worse; then draw a petal looping back into the problem. If it is genuinely helpful, extend the arrow out.

It's called a "flower" because the arrows (things that we do) that flow out from the center (the pain or distress) often loop back like petals. It's called a "vicious flower" in the same sense that we use the term *vicious circle*—it describes how these petals can make things worse and become ingrained. If all this seems a bit abstract, look at Sophia's vicious flower, which gets activated when she feels criticized.

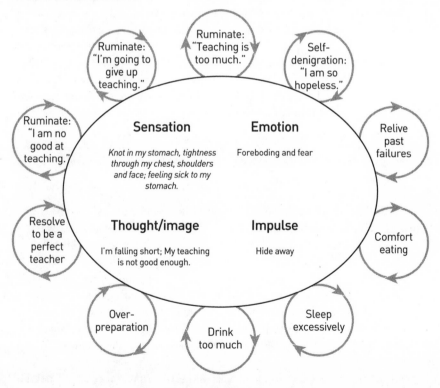

Sophia's inner critic.

What We Can Learn from the Vicious Flower

Stand back and look at what happens to you when you're stressed. What do you notice? What can you learn about how you cope in these situations? Here are some of the most common and important lessons people describe:

1. Not only can you understand stress (as you saw in Chapter 5), but these moments when a stimulus starts to trigger reactivity can become an early warning system.

2. We don't like to feel bad. It automatically and understandably triggers reactivity. As you've already seen, this link in the formation of a vicious flower is key; it is what sets off trying to fix how we feel. It's the point at which the "first arrow" can easily turn into the "second arrow" or more than likely a whole volley of arrows! We don't like it, we don't want it, we want it to go away, so understandably we try to fix it. These second arrows curve around and come back at us, forming the petals of a vicious flower.

3. The strategies you noticed probably fall into two broad groups. First, avoidance—trying to get away or avoid the situation and bad feelings. It's amazing how many ways we can dream up to run away! Second, trying to think our way out of the problem. We can find ourselves endlessly analyzing the situation, ruminating about the past, worrying about the future, having debates with ourselves, rehearsing memories over and over. Of course, our amazing ability to learn and problem-solve can help us out of tricky situations. But there are many situations where thinking our way out of problems just entangles us and doesn't help.

> SOPHIA: *Looking at my "inner critic" vicious flower, now I can see that the petals in the bottom half are mostly ways of running away and those in the top half are ways of trying to think my way out of it.*

4. It's likely you're using all these things for good reasons. But the important question you're asking yourself now is "Does this coping strategy serve me?" Yes, it may make me feel better, but what about in the bigger picture? Is it helpful or a "second arrow that loops back to make a petal of your vicious flower"?

> SOPHIA: *The other day I was in the kitchen, I'd had a difficult day, I was feeling antsy, and I was eating ice cream straight out of the tub with a large spoon when my daughter came in with her matter-of-fact "Mum, you're eating your feelings again. How do they taste?" I had to laugh. Our kids can be truth tellers; she was right of course.*

Comfort eating is a good example of a second arrow that makes up the petal in the vicious flower. But eating is of course how we fuel ourselves, even eating ice cream! I remember in the final weeks of my father's life his diet involved mostly ice cream—not only did he enjoy it, but the caloric content helped him at a time that the cancer was emaciating him. With weeks to live, no one was going to say, "That's not good for you; you'll put on weight." Instead, eating a lot of ice cream gave him some joy at a very difficult time. So, it is not the strategy itself that makes it a petal or an arrow leading out; it's why we're doing it and whether its effects serve us or keep us locked into unhelpful habits.

SOPHIA: My "inner critic" vicious flower has quite a few petals. Every one of them is sort of familiar, like a go-to way of coping. But all of them, if I stand back, don't really challenge my shaky sense of being good enough. In fact, they mostly make it so that my sense of self-worth relies on people praising me and not criticizing me. It keeps my inner critic in place, rather than allowing it to be exposed for what it is, a house of cards.

5. Recognizing your patterns of reactivity is the first step in creating a sense of possibility that you can change. These are patterns you can step out of.

SOPHIA: Sometimes I comfort-eat, take to my bed, and drink too much. I know that sometimes doing these things is okay. But if I do this all the time (wincing uncomfortably), I will become obese, lonely, a problem drinker, and get unhealthy.

PRACTICE:	Using the Three-Step Breathing Space to Recognize Patterns of Reactivity

You've started using the Breathing Space (go back and reread page 60 in Chapter 3 if that would be a helpful). A quick reminder. The Breathing Space is a simple way to pause and recognize what's happening in any given moment. It can be particularly helpful in moments of difficulty, stress, and reactivity. Watching your reactive mind in full flow can be a brilliant teacher. Maybe the next time you experience a vicious flower taking form, try taking a Breathing Space.

SOPHIA: Yesterday I asked a colleague for feedback, and when they didn't reply immediately, my mind did its worst. There I was, in the grip of my inner critic. So, I did a Breathing Space. If I'm honest, I felt terrible, hopeless, stuck. It didn't help at all; it made it worse in a way. What familiar territory, the knot in my stomach, reliving past failures, being so down on myself and reaching for the cookie jar! How many years have I lived with this critic? When it takes hold, I literally feel locked in, trapped.

SAM: I couldn't help but crack a smile. I did it on the bus on the way home. A tough shift at work, one of my patients had died, we hadn't been able to get a handle on her pain, it was brutal. And just when I thought this can't get worse, there was a pointless management meeting after the shift. Managers can be so bureaucratic and heartless.

So, there I am on the bus, just wanting to vanish into my phone. Played a game, decided to take a ninja—that's what I call your Breathing Spaces. I looked up, and it was insane, almost everyone on the bus was glued to their phone, totally zoned out from the world. I had to smile; it felt like we're all in this together, part of the same human family, you know. Each of us just trying to do our best, finding our escapes and bits of happiness where we can. I am not going to lie; I went back to my phone, but with a smile on my face.

LING: *I had a meeting with my boss. His style is so grating. I get more and more irritated and usually leave the meeting in a bad mood. I tried doing a Breathing Space before the meeting and said to myself, "Try keeping 50% of your attention in your body during the meeting." I was still irritated and noticed my shoulders tightened, my jaw contracted, my breathing was shallower. Not nice. But recognizing it stopped my irritability from spiraling into a foul mood. I was still irritated, but I wasn't going to let it ruin my day. I was quietly proud of myself, and at the end of the day, when we were finishing up, a colleague who I get on with quite well said, "What's going on with you, Ling? You seem different."*

The Breathing Space helped Sophia, Sam, and Ling step back and see their reactive mind in action. This pause and shift in perspective is a teacher. We may not like what we see, but at least we have a chance to learn. In Sophia's case, how ingrained these habits are. In Sam's case, how what he does is what most people do. Ling could see a very familiar set of feelings and sensations, and that recognition broke the chain of reactivity.

The Ancient Oak:
You Can't Step in the Same River Twice

In the 6th century B.C.E., Heraclitus, the Greek philosopher, is thought to have written something along the lines of "Into the same rivers we step and do not step, we are and are not." He was saying that on the one hand we and rivers can be named and described. I have an identity, but on the other hand I am also constantly changing moment by moment. The same is true of a river; it has a name, but as the water flows it changes all the time. *These changes define a river, and they define us.* If the river wasn't constantly changing, with moving water, and all the beings that exist in and around it, it would be something else, a lake, a lagoon, a creek. If I wasn't in flux, my body and mind, then I wouldn't be alive.

So, when you turn to your experience in a three-step Breathing Space, you're noting, often using words, what you are in that moment, and if you can stay curious and open, you'll come to see that there are myriad different experiences that make up your life, and yet you're still you.

> ## PRACTICE: Mindful Walking Revisited
>
> Mindful walking was introduced in Chapter 3, but many people say it is a great way to ground themselves when they are reactive. That's my experience too. The word *grounding* is interesting; it literally means connecting with the ground, and when you walk you ground through your feet. It takes us away from our heads, full of thoughts, and even our torso, full of sensations and feelings. Our feet in contact with the ground, rooted even, and our legs moving very intentionally, can be very steadying and soothing. A bit like with the Breathing Space, here are two things to try.
>
> 1. More than likely, there is a place you walk every day. Is there a path you could make your "walking path"? A reminder to "come to," walk with awareness, and if possible, even slow down? It doesn't need to be a big deal; you're walking a route you walk anyway but using it to ground yourself.
> 2. Can you use walking with awareness intentionally, in moments of difficulty or stress, at times you know you might otherwise be reactive? At a time when it might be helpful to step out of your thoughts and feelings and ground yourself?

SOPHIA: *I'm retired now, but when I was a teacher I made the walk from my classroom to the front door of the school my walking path. I was usually heading to greet a child or parent, and it was a chance to just settle myself and let go of where I was coming from, just be in my walking body and then bring to mind whoever I was about to meet.*

Taking It Further:
Getting More Skillful at Bringing Awareness to Difficulties

Stress and difficulty are a part of life, so we must learn to cope with them. Bringing awareness to difficulties isn't without risk, so I want to introduce some ways you can navigate stress and difficulties with skill, care, and wisdom.

Grounding and Anchoring

You've started to explore different ways of gathering your mind. You've hopefully developed a range of ways to gather and steady yourself. You've also started to explore different anchors for different circumstances (Chapter 2, pages 43–44, and Chapter 3, pages 60–61). When you're feeling calm and steady, this might be the subtlest of sensations of breathing in the nostrils or across the lips. When you're feeling very agitated or sleepy, it may be the soles of your feet or your hands. Sometimes things happen that are very upsetting or overwhelming. At these times you may need to physically move—your anchor here is your body moving, such as the changing sensations in the feet and legs.

Some people need an anchor outside their body. This can be through touch, listening, or fixing your gaze on something. Sometimes you need an anchor outside of the body, like something in the distance you can look at or a sound you can settle your attention on. As this becomes more familiar, something you have confidence in, you can play with moving between different anchors, including in the body and outside the body.

> LING: *Driving is a time when I often start thinking about tricky stuff in my life. I use the steering wheel as an anchor. I tune in to my grip on the wheel and the movements as I drive. Sometimes I play with moving my attention between something outside me, like the steering wheel, and inside me, like my breath, which maybe starts off quite shallow and sort of tight, but often eases off.*

Our Bodies as a Sanctuary

Our minds can be goal-oriented and trip into overthinking. That's why awareness of our body can be so useful. As you've already learned, the body is not only a possible anchor but also has so much to say, if only you will listen.

> SOPHIA: *When I started teaching, during each term and teaching year I would get more and more exhausted. I was so busy I barely noticed. I pushed through. Looking back, now I can see that I was sleeping less and less well, drinking more each evening, exercising less. When I saw my parents, they'd say, "Sophia, are you okay? You look tired." They could see it, and I couldn't, because I wasn't paying attention. Teaching is hard. The kids show up each day, and you have to show up too to teach them, set and mark their work, do all the pastoral stuff, meet with parents. But like I said, I started to use the walk from my classroom to the front as a time to check in. I'd listen to my body a bit more.*

You're starting to become *familiar with how your body and mind are reacting to difficulties.* This may be contraction, heat, intensity, discomfort. It may be in your face, throat, shoulders, chest, belly, arms, and hands. It may be a sense of the whole body being agitated. You've started to see how reactivity plays out for you, maybe even given it a name—"my inner critic," "Skinny Sam," "my black dog."

Moving Toward, Moving Away, and Tuning Out

Our minds will naturally orient toward some things and away from others. Some of this is deep in our biology, learned through our evolutionary history—an automatic alerting to threat—and some we have learned in our lives. Mindfulness is not about having to accept everything passively or stare down difficulties. Rather, it is about knowing when to move toward or away from things, be that sensations in our bodies, habits of mind, relationships, jobs.

> **The Ancient Oak and the Barefoot Professor:**
> **The "Guest House"**
>
> **The Ancient Oak:** The 13th-century poet Jalāl ad-Dīn Muhammad Rūmī wrote a poem likening being human to being a guest house. We have all these visitors, some we really like, others we don't, some maybe scare us, others we don't understand. He invites us to welcome and honor them all, because there may be something we can learn from them.
>
> It's a poem that can be so helpful if we use it wisely. A guest house needs a strong door with a good lock. We choose to whom and when to open it. Sometimes we keep the door locked, maybe talk to someone while they stay outside. When we do welcome someone in, we also choose how long they stay, whether to serve them a drink, a meal, or offer them a place to stay for a while. Sometimes a guest might become a friend.
>
> Rūmī's invitation to welcome and honor all guests is an active and discerning process, not passive, nor reckless.
>
> **The Barefoot Professor:** Living organisms also actively move toward and away from different stimuli. Amoeba will move depending on the concentration of chemicals in and around them. Some flowers will open to and follow the sun through the day and then close at night. Our minds similarly move naturally toward what is pleasant and away from what is unpleasant.

Protective mindfulness involves recognizing a pain, dark thoughts, or sadness—the first arrow. And then making good choices about what you choose to allow into awareness or, conversely, turn away.

> LING: *Sometimes I feel sad for no good reason. My reflex at these times is to duvet-dive and ruminate—the same old, same old, "Why do I feel sad?" "Will this never end?" I see the sadness as the first arrow, and the duvet dive and rumination are second arrows. Yes, firing them is a reflex, and I am slowly but surely learning it is a choice.*

Grounding and anchoring help us here. If you're grounded and anchored, you can explore this idea of moving toward and away from difficulties. You can bring an interest to where the sensations are, where they are strongest, where they begin and end, how they change moment by moment. If you're feeling less steady or it's too intense, come back to your anchor and let the sensations, as best you can, move into the background. You can know when something is okay to look at and be with, when it isn't, and when it's best to distract yourself or even to tune out altogether. For example, in very traumatic situations, parts of our mind can shut down by themselves, to protect us from being overwhelmed. This means you can do what is needed.

> SOPHIA: *When my mother was in palliative care in a hospice in the final stages of heart failure, I tried to be with her as much as possible. I had a sense that if I could stay present in these moments there was a lot I could learn. The uncertainty, unpleasantness of shortness of breath, fear of dying, loss of dignity, tiredness, crumbling boundaries between living and dying, present and absent, here and not here—it was a lot for any mind to cope with, and sometimes I needed to turn away and even shut down completely. I trusted this. My sister and I took turns, so we could take breaks.*

Attitude, or Lens of Mindfulness

The poet Emily Dickinson wrote a poem, "Tell the truth but tell it slant," where she invites the reader to approach the truth at a "slant," so that it reveals itself gradually rather than blinding us. She is pointing to approaching difficulties with care, slowly.

> MOHAMMED: *At college some coaches really only cared about winning games. We were dispensable athletes there to help them win, easily replaceable. I remember being asked to play when my back pain was bad, and they told me to just play through it, be strong, and if need be, the team doctor could give me a steroid shot and I could take painkillers during the game. I did, and it really messed up my back. I kind of knew my body needed something else, but I listened to the coaches because I believed they had my destiny in their hands. I wish I had been wise and brave enough to listen to my body and not to the coaches.*
>
> *Since I retired from sports, I have had to learn to live with the pain, and this has taken a lot of time, not fighting it, or trying to push through it. The single biggest thing that has helped has been learning to recognize it, give it some space, and sometimes I even choose to put it center stage. Instead of trusting coaches or team doctors, I trust myself; I listen to what my body is trying to say. What makes this easier is when I listen as if I were listening to a good friend or to my children. My son fell off his bike the other day, cut up his lip, and a tooth was knocked out. He was white as a sheet, crying, and somehow I was able to scoop him up and console him—"It's okay, that was scary, you're being really brave." I try to bring the same care to my pain now, and that attitude of scooping up, caring, and courage is what makes it possible.*

Titration

Imagine exposing yourself to all the bad news in the world; it would be overwhelming, very upsetting, and why on earth would you want to do that? With our minds this sort of approach more than likely would not just cause pain but could also be damaging.

Over time you can calibrate the levels at which you can work with difficulties—that feeling is manageable, that one is overwhelming—right now. That pain is tolerable, but this one is not. Gathering and anchoring our attention is foundational for this work. So is learning how to soothe yourself.

The Barefoot Professor and the Ancient Oak: Titration

The Barefoot Professor: Your liver has many functions, processing key substances, managing your fuel by converting glycogen to glucose and storing extra glucose by converting it to glycogen and managing toxins. Your attention and awareness are doing much the same thing. We can borrow the idea of "titration" from chemistry. We need the right amount of glucose or toxins to function; so too we need to titrate the right amount of experiences, pleasant, rewarding and challenging to function.

The Ancient Oak: If we took a pinch of salt and put it in a thimble of water, it would be aversive to drink. But take the same pinch and put it in a large enough pitcher and it becomes possible to drink it and barely taste the salt. Put it in a huge lake, and you wouldn't taste the salt at all. The same is true with body sensations, emotions, impulses, and thoughts. If our attention is consumed by the sensations, like salt in a thimble, they are overpowering and unpalatable. But if we stand back and hold them in much more expansive awareness, we can see them clearly and have more of a chance of being able to work with them.

If you're tired, there is a lot going on, you don't feel in great shape—this is a time to take care of yourself and not take on any more than you can manage. If on the other hand you're feeling stable and steady, have a sense of being well resourced, this might be a time you can take on a bit more, let in more, work with more intense experiences.

MOHAMMED: *My back pain is like a living being. Some days it whispers quietly; other days it's a raging beast that threatens to consume me. The quiet days are easy; the raging beast is not. I started to get curious in the quiet days. Where were the sensations? What were they whispering? This wasn't without risk, because turning toward them often made them noisier. But it helps me fear the pain less, made me able to stay curious and keep asking, "What will help in this moment?" Sometimes it's acceptance, sometimes it's movement, sometimes it's a painkiller, and sometimes nothing works. What I have learned over the years is that more than likely I am going to have to live with this for the rest of my life. That is a terrifying thought. A friend had a motorcycle accident and couldn't live with the pain from the injuries he sustained and eventually took his life. I get that, how pain could become so unbearable. So, if I am going to live with it, I need to do everything I can to resource myself to manage the okay and difficult days and survive the terrible days.*

Mindfulness builds your capacity, so you are better able to work with difficulties. You can hold and manage more. In the next chapter you'll do more on building your capacity to work with difficulties by cultivating attitudes such as curiosity, kindness, care, and courage.

Recognizing Our Patterns of Reactivity in Real Life, for Life

The vicious flower exercise is not something you do once; it's something to use in many areas of your life, and for life. The ways you've learned to react are often habits that more than likely have strong roots. It takes practice to recognize each time a vicious flower plays out in your life.

The Vicious Flower Revisited

What one thing tells you that a vicious flower is playing out—that you are in the grip of reactivity?

In your vicious flower, is there a strong signal that you can trust and use that tells you, ah, here it is playing out again? It may be a bodily sensation, like Sophia's sinking feeling in her gut. Or it may be a powerful impulse, as for example Ling describes it—"a duvet dive." Irritability is a hallmark for Mohammed.

The more you can see your unhelpful habits playing out by, for example, using Breathing Spaces, the more you can stand back from them. Each of the elements of the vicious flower can be seen afresh over and over. You can learn to see the sensations, moods, impulses, and thoughts that trigger reactivity, just as they are.

MOHAMMED: *I mentioned I am not proud of getting irritable. But after the kids were born it got worse and my wife and I had some couples therapy. It was eye opening—I didn't know how to argue. What I thought was me keeping the peace to her was sulking. The therapist explained that going into myself can be a sign of trouble ahead—she called it stonewalling. We needed to find a better way to talk about things we didn't see the same way.*

In an argument, just before withdrawing, there may well be fear. Or anger, and an impulse to hurt the other person. You can see the ways you try to avoid and fix what you don't like or can't tolerate. Withdrawing keeps others at arm's length, keeps us safe. It can also be punitive, a powerful indirect way of expressing anger. The more you practice, the better you can see all the elements of the vicious flower, but also each of the links in the chain of reactivity.

> MOHAMMED: *My wife and I discussed how in these moments we would call out what was happening, and because withdrawing is what I do instinctively, I could ask her to give me some time. Just naming it and taking a pause, including a Breathing Space, to see it clearly and shift perspective, was already a big step in the right direction. I love my wife, and the last thing I want to do is hurt her.*

This slowing down and seeing, especially if you can hold your values in mind, brings into focus what is helpful and what isn't. Stonewalling, punitiveness, avoiding conflict rarely serve us or indeed anyone else.

The Vicious Flower's Roots

The wanting, craving, and striving described in Chapter 5 is fertile ground for the vicious flower to grow some deep roots. Like roots, we've each, through our upbringing, and through the inevitable trial and error of our lives, learned various beliefs and rules for living.

> MOHAMMED: *My parents had very fixed roles. My father ran a small home appliance repair business and was out of the house most of the day six days a week. My mother was a matriarch, and her dominion was the home and us kids. They stuck to these roles, and I don't really remember ever much seeing them argue. Like any family, we had lots of unspoken rules. Growing up, one of the main ones was that arguing was not a good thing. My wife is super comfortable calling out issues, including an argument, if need be, and in the early days of our marriage I had no idea how to handle that—my rule was stay in our lanes, and there would no reason to argue. You can imagine, this really annoys her.*

> SOPHIA: *"I need to be a perfect teacher, or I am not good enough" is a rule that has dictated so much of my life. I got a message from my parents and school that being successful academically was essential, that if I wasn't I would fail in life. If I think about it, every place I have studied or worked has propped up my unrelenting standards. This has made this root system a bit like the bamboo in my garden—it's taken over. I was in therapy for a while, and I realized this root system was even deeper. I have this inescapable sense of unworthiness that I've picked up from a sense of always being compared, unfavorably, with my sister, with other teachers. My first serious boyfriend also used to*

gaslight me. I didn't even notice it at the time, maybe because he was saying what I also said to myself. I gaslit myself as much as he did for years.

When your rules for living don't serve you, maybe they need to change. Our emotions evolved to help us survive. They can signal that something important is happening. Shame, guilt, anger, irritation, sadness, surprise, contempt— these are all powerful communications. Each will likely have associated thoughts and stories. If emotions are particularly powerful, or seem to have a patterning or regularity, it is worth getting curious and looking under the surface to see if they reveal our rules for living. Very often rules for living have to do with worth, lovability, and our sense of being able to make a difference in our lives. Often, they come as "if–then" statements. Here are some common examples: "If I get criticized, it means I am no good." "If I am vulnerable with people, they'll hurt me." "If I am not in control, something bad will happen." "If I don't do things perfectly, people will think I am useless." "If I show people the real me, they'll reject me." And of course, we also have rules for how others should behave and what we think the world should be like. It's interesting to start exploring the rules you use. If your exploration can be playful, or at least kind, it makes it more possible to be honest with yourself.

> What are your rules for living that don't serve you? What would a more helpful rule look like?

SOPHIA: *I remember a teacher who everyone loved, and thought was by far the coolest teacher at the school. One day he came into the class with his characteristic style and charisma, picked up a chair, turned it around to sit on it back to front, and slid off the back of the chair—not a slick move at all. But he laughed at himself just as hard as the kids laughed at him, and he didn't try to cover it up. Everyone loved him even more for showing his vulnerability and his honesty. Even though I've retired, we're still friends— he's still cool, vulnerable, and honest. If I'd fallen off a chair like that in front of a class, I would have been mortified. I guess his rule is something like: "I can make mistakes, people will still like me." My rule was "If I make any kind of mistake, it means I am going to be found out and fired."*

The Vicious Flower's Ecosystem

I have described the vicious flower as something we create in our body–mind. But they are first created by what is happening in our wider world—living in relentless poverty, a home environment that is unsafe, being exposed to or witnessing various forms of abuse, being bullied at school, parents with unrelenting standards, working in a harmful work environment or being in a coercive or abusive relationship. These are conditions where helplessness, fear, abuse, and feeling not good enough are normal, understandable reactions. And it is where strong associations and rules for living are first developed. It helps to see reactivity as understandable, helpful even, in these circumstances. You can't erase your history, but you also don't need to replicate it in your present or, even if your past wasn't harmful, stick with a situation now that is harmful. Recognizing reactivity, using your emotions as an alerting system, you can start to see how your history and your life circumstances now powerfully shape your experience, rules for living, and values.

You've seen how and why unhelpful ways of thinking and behaving can become habits—like a vicious flower. Unchecked, they can multiply. I had a dog that was in a fight with a larger brown bulldog and was badly hurt. Not surprisingly he developed a fear of large brown bulldogs. He would bark at them; he was a terrier and had a strong bark. I guess he figured, "I'll scare them before they can get to me." But over time this behavior generalized to all large brown dogs, then to medium-size dogs. Later in his life as his hearing and vision deteriorated, he barked at all moving objects! The same can happen with us: a vicious flower can generalize to new situations and take in new forms—you can become reactive in more and more situations. Mohammed's fear of conflict and rule, "if I stay in my lane, there will be no conflict," was learned at home, but generalized to school, his relationship with sports coaches, and his wife.

> Has your reactivity spread to different areas of your life? If so, maybe a rule for living or core belief, perhaps around worth or lovability, underlies all of this?

LING: *Before I was taken into care, I lived with my biological father and mother. He was a man who was so filled with rage. It was like walking on eggshells. My mother coped with his rage by drinking; she was often out of it. Living in my family was like living in an earthquake zone, with constant tremors of anger, fear, bewilderment, lies, and confusion. I eventually was taken into care.*

Not surprisingly I am fearful of relationships. I live in fear and can be haunted by nightmares. I often get drawn into endless rumination: "Why me? Did I bring this on myself? Should I have done something differently?" Weird as it sounds, as a child I blamed myself. "What was wrong with me that my father got angry?" When I moved into foster and then residential care I hunkered down, but trust, fear, blame, why me, it all simply played out over and over again with peers and foster parents. Any encounter with an authority figure could trigger waves of terror and helplessness and cast me back into the past. Even shows of love would make me suspicious and hostile. This was the only way I knew how to stay safe.

When I was in my 30s, two women came forward to say my father had abused them, physically, sexually, and emotionally. He had remarried and they were the

*children of his second wife. He was charged on 21 counts and pleaded not guilty to all
of them. I sat through the six-week trial, recognizing that much of what had happened
to them had also happened to me. It brought up guilt, shame, and anger. I told some of
my closest friends. One of them came to court with me. It was hard to sit through, but
also a relief that he was found guilty on all charges. The trial raised all sorts of issues
for me, and I got some therapy. It helped me to make sense of what had happened, and
I reached out to the other women who were abused by him. I can't say I am cured or
anything. What happened is always going to be horrible, but I see it now as a scar that
I can touch with care, rather than an open wound I didn't even dare to look at. This
means I don't live my life in continual shame, anger, and reactivity. My mindfulness
practice is a place that resources me.*

If reactivity takes hold of more and more parts of your life, it becomes how
you define yourself and others, and that can start to become your life. For Ling
mistrust had generalized to relationships with men and her work, with a rule
for living that to trust people is to open oneself up to being abused.

Recognizing and Disarming Reactivity throughout Life

Difficulties are part and parcel of life, and you will, like everyone, develop a
whole repertoire of ways of coping. Some of these are helpful, and others may
have served you in the past but now lock you into problems and unhappiness.
You can learn to see what does and doesn't work for you and to recognize
unhelpful reactivity, so it doesn't come to rule your life. Geological pressure
transforms silt to limestone. Extreme heat and pressure deep in the earth's core
can even transform organic material into diamonds. Strange as it may sound,
difficulties may well turn out not to be hindrances, but the making of us. But
all of this takes patience, applied effort, and time. Seeing things as they are and
knowing why they are as they are are important steps along the way. Once you
have recognized your reactivity, you have the chance to respond wisely. We'll
turn to this in the next few chapters.

Befriending Our Minds

Mindfulness is awareness shaped by friendliness.

W hat makes a good friend? These are some of the qualities that people often mention: "genuine," "trustworthy," "kind," "good listener," "accepts me as I am," "fun," "has my back," "makes an effort," and "makes me feel good about myself." Can you imagine going through every moment of your life accompanied by someone like this? Well, it's quite possible to cultivate this kind of friendship, because you can befriend your own mind. In this chapter, we'll explore the idea that awareness only becomes mindfulness when it is lit, colored, and shaped by friendliness.

You've explored the idea that you can intentionally gather your mind and anchor your attention. You can come home to your body. You can access different ways of knowing and being. You can use all of this to recognize and step back from reactivity. What we'll move to now is how to befriend your mind by cultivating attitudes such as friendly curiosity, appreciation, and care. You'll learn how these attitudes can be woven into your practice and life, helping you both to work with reactivity and to savor and build all that is good in your life.

Exploring the Prevailing Landscape of Your Own Mind

This exploration starts with the question "What is the prevailing landscape of our hearts and minds?"

SOPHIA: *When I was a teacher, I had a reputation as someone who didn't suffer fools gladly. When I started meditating, I realized that I applied this maxim to myself, often in quite a harsh way. It is no surprise I was always trying to be perfect to avoid being found wanting, or worse still a fool, by of all people, myself.*

SAM: *I prefer to not keep things on the down-low when it comes to what's going in there (pointing to his head, and then grins, also pointing to his heart). That's why I'm all about gaming when I am not working. I guess if I'm honest, I can be a bit remote, cut off.*

MOHAMMED: *Years as an elite athlete ingrained in me this constant striving to improve. More, better. Always, more, better. It's exhausting.*

LING: *I used to think my husband was my soul mate, that we were destined to be together. But he became ever more controlling as time went on, and when the kids were born, he just couldn't handle it. He tried to control everything I did as a mother, as a wife, he made me give up work, and I lost touch with most of my friends. My world got smaller and smaller and started to feel like a prison. The irony is that when I eventually left him, it was almost worse, because I had lost my confidence. When I started meditating, it dawned on me that I was still imprisoned by a sense of being useless. A friend told me that the Chinese symbols for soul mate—灵魂伴侣—mean literally to know oneself, that is to say, to be my own soul mate. That's what I'm working on.*

If you were to describe the normal qualities of your mind, what would they be? I know this is like asking a fish, "What are you swimming around in?" The fish has no idea; the water all around it simply exists. Learning to observe your mind starts to reveal your mind's qualities. But here is the good news: This is where you can start to train the qualities that make your mind a good friend.

Curiosity, Kindness, Appreciation, and Care

The shift from turning away to turning toward your life with attitudes of curiosity, kindness, appreciation, and care is one of the most important changes you can make.

Curiosity

Curiosity means being open to and interested in what is happening in the outside world and in our minds and bodies. Curiosity can mean letting go, as best we can, of assumptions and seeing things afresh, with a playful, childlike interest. It can also be deeply inquiring, where we explore something thoroughly. This means also seeing the parts that are harder to see for all sorts of reasons, such as that they're hidden, or we feel they're not as acceptable. Or it can be like a scientific endeavor, where we ask questions and set out to answer them systematically. Dialed all the way up, interest can be a sense of awe.

Benjamin Zander, a talented, energetic, and charismatic music conductor and teacher, is mentoring a 15-year-old musician. The boy is playing a Bach composition, and it's plain how hard he is trying to do well. At a certain moment he makes a barely noticeable mistake, and if you pay close attention, you can see a tiny grimace cross his face. From this moment on he seems to shift from playing the piece to trying to get to the end without making any more mistakes. Afterward Zander says in a very matter-of-fact way, "You made a mistake halfway through." The boy looks horrified, but Zander smiles kindly, and with real care and enthusiasm goes on to say, "When you make a mistake, try to respond with 'Isn't that fascinating?'" This is a profound shift of attitude. It is natural for us to contract and be self-critical if something goes wrong. But for this young musician the contraction made his playing procedural. Benjamin Zander is suggesting that we respond to mistakes with curiosity because this opens us up to learning and growing.

The prevailing climate of our minds will be how we meet the moments of each day. Meeting these moments with friendly curiosity, maybe even with a stance of "Isn't that fascinating," makes it possible to be playful and creative.

Kindness

Curiosity opens our awareness. Kindness or friendliness goes further and imbues our awareness with qualities of interest and care. It doesn't say, "I'll be friendly only to this and not to that." It is unconditional. It involves turning toward all our bodily sensations, moods, thoughts, and experiences, whether they are pleasant, unpleasant, or neutral, with interest and kindness. It doesn't mean looking to change anything. Instead, befriending our minds means relating to all that is already happening with kindness. It involves trusting that over time this will become the shape of our minds.

Kindness is not soft or weak, as Charlotte Brontë puts it in her novel *Jane Eyre*. It is "far more potent than force."

> SAM: *Going out used to mess with my head big time. I'm an introvert who likes people and going out. But I used to get this nagging voice in my head telling me if I went out no one would want to chat to me, that I'd be too different, maybe people would make fun of me—you know, the whole thing blah, blah, blah. The voice in my head? Picture a big burly man, straight out of a nightclub bouncer scene. Turns out, he reminded me of a soccer coach from back in the day, when I was a kid who I kinda liked but was low-key scared of. Ex-military, did security at nightclubs, father of a neighborhood kid. Somehow, I started talking back to this man in my head, and it turns out he was just trying to help me out. We became good friends. Now when he pipes up, it's all about encouraging me to go out, make friends, and just enjoy myself. He's like "It's okay, I've got your back," and "You're looking good." He has my back, and it's a game-changer.*

Appreciation

Friendly curiosity opens us up to our lives. It makes wholehearted enjoyment possible, be that of music, the feeling of the sun's warmth on our face, someone we care about smiling, a good meal, or all that is right with our body in any given moment. If we're curious and open, these moments are available throughout the day. You have already started to develop the attitudes of appreciation, joy, and gratitude. (Go back to Chapter 4 if you need a reminder.) I hope this has shown you that contentment and joy are much more than passing moments of happiness. They are a quality of mind and a way of being. It is part of the landscape of your mind. You become more inclined to notice and savor good things. You start to deliberately seek them out, and they become who you are and characterize your life. When appreciation is fully integrated into your life, it becomes enduring contentment.

Care

Just as curiosity opens us up to the good, it also opens us up to painful and difficult experiences. This is where care comes in. It enables us to recognize pain, be open and accepting of it, and respond in ways that ease the suffering. We have all experienced moments of feeling moved by pain, distress, and suffering, whether our own or others. This can be tending to a sick child, witnessing an elderly relative becoming increasingly frail, experiencing physical pain, watching a tired parent cope with an infant's tantrum, or having worries about what is happening in the wider world. Pain and suffering are part of the universal human experience. Compassion is deeply caring about, connecting with, and responding to pain.

The Ancient Oak and the Barefoot Professor: Compassion

The Ancient Oak: The roots in Latin (*compati*) are *to suffer with*, which has this sense of resonating with and being alongside suffering. Contemplative traditions tend to emphasize compassion as a key value and practice. Typically, these traditions invite moving beyond self-centered concerns and responding compassionately to others. They provide practices that support this, be that prayer, meditation, contemplations, or reading.

The Barefoot Professor: That's interesting, because you can trace the science of compassion in earliest evolutionary psychology to Charles Darwin. He observed that in many highly social species, compassion acts to make the group cohesive. This group cohesion provides an evolutionary advantage. Developmental psychologists have shown that infants can sense distress in others, but initially can't distinguish it from their own distress and so get upset. Only later, when they develop theory of mind, knowing that others think and feel too, does compassion become more sophisticated.

    Also, it's hardwired. When we act with kindness or care, certain sensory–motor–emotion areas and networks are activated, and there is evidence that vividly imagining these situations activates these areas. This suggests that we can, with our extraordinary capacity for imagination, prime these neural networks and body systems. There is also evidence that the more we imagine specific instances, use imagery, and enrich the image and experience, the more beneficial this might be. It's practicing in safety a skill that we can then put into action in our lives.

This suggests the capacity for compassion is both deep in our nature and something we can learn.

Cultivating the Friendship between You and Your Mind

We started this chapter with the qualities of a good friend: "genuine," "trustworthy," "kind," "good listener," "accepts me as I am," "fun," "has my back," "makes an effort," and "makes me feel good about myself." Some friends are fun to be around and with others we feel safe; perhaps there is someone who is a good listener and another who always knows the right thing to say. No two friendships are the same. We tend to go to different friends for different things. Finally, we have to work at friendships.

In the same way, I am suggesting that befriending your mind involves cultivating a particular set of 10 attitudes, which you go to for different reasons, at different times, and which together help you befriend your mind. Like any friendship, befriending your mind starts with being interested in and appreciative of one another. Once you are open and appreciative of your mind, with all its quirks and qualities, you're adding being kind, and at times of difficulty being caring. To this I'd like to add trust, patience, courage, equanimity, and letting go. All of this requires just the right amount of effort, not too much, or it becomes striving, not too little or you flounder.

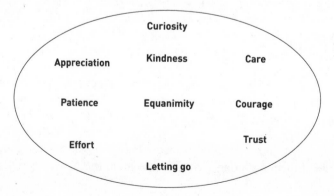

Ten Attitudes of Mindfulness

Why 10? It's not a magic number, but there is a body of evidence that these 10 qualities support us in our lives. And importantly, there are established ways to cultivate them, both through mindfulness practices and in our everyday lives.

The Ancient Oak and the Barefoot Professor:
Mindfulness Practice as Cultivation

The Ancient Oak: In Buddhist psychology the Pāli and Sanskrit term *bhāvanaā* means to cultivate or bring into existence. In Tibetan (translation, *sgom*) it's familiarization, and in Chinese they bring in the idea of practice (*xiuxing* 修行). But these ideas can also be traced to the Greeks, who spoke about training (*meletē*) and exercise (*askēsis*). These ideas of training go beyond Eastern traditions and reside in Christian, Muslim, and many other religious and contemplative traditions.

The Barefoot Professor: Many people have compared mindfulness training to physical exercise. Physical exercise can improve our strength, flexibility, and cardiovascular fitness. Different physical regimes are used for these different outcomes, resistance training for strength, yoga for flexibility and exercise that increases heart rate for cardiovascular fitness. Exercise has to be matched to the person—and if it isn't, it can cause harm. Mindfulness practice has many parallels. Mindfulness practice needs first to do no harm. Different mindfulness practices produce different effects, training needs to be personalized, and what works for one person won't work for another. In the same way that aerobic exercise builds cardiovascular fitness, so mindfulness practices can prioritize attention to develop focus. The difference between mindfulness practice and physical exercise is that much of the learning in mindfulness doesn't just ebb away if we stop practicing. Mindfulness practice is all about learning to relate differently to our bodies and minds, and much of what we learn can't really be forgotten. We may forget to practice, or get caught up again in old habits, but our ability to bring awareness to our experience and relate to it differently will always be there, available to us. And we don't have to go to the gym or anywhere special to practice; we can practice in our everyday lives.

The word *cultivation* is perfect to describe the work of mindfulness in real life, for life. The meaning many people think of is how we cultivate crops, forests, or a garden, using what we know and the natural conditions of climate, soil, sunlight, temperature, and so on. What develops is a product of our work and the natural conditions. And it takes time, like planting seeds and then taking care of them until they grow and mature in their own way and time. A garden might take many years to become mature. This is also how you cultivate attitudes of mind, using many of the same ideas: intentionally, creating the right conditions, adapting over time, and then patiently allowing the process to unfold. You'll explore next *how* you can befriend your mind and body, first with mindfulness practices and then in everyday life.

Befriending Your Mind through Mindfulness Practices

The mindfulness practices introduced so far have been mainly about bringing your attention to your breath or your body. You may have noticed an encouragement to do this with interest and friendliness, which means that you have already started this work of reshaping your mind by inclining it toward an attitude of friendly interest.

> SAM: *The first time I dipped my toes into meditation, I had this annoying itch on my forearm. Psoriasis means I'm no stranger to itchiness. But as I'm trying to meditate, I get this crazy urge to scratch and my mind goes on a wild ride: "I hate having psoriasis. People will see my skin and think I'm a weirdo and not want to know me. I really want to scratch this itch, but I know if I do, I'll aggravate the psoriasis and break out in an awful rash, and that will make it worse." I'm basically giving myself a hard time. I decide to experiment. What if I deliberately resist scratching? At first, the urge cranks up to eleven. It's almost unbearable—I catch my hand moving toward that itch! When I bring a friendly interest to it, though, it creates a little space. Time enough to see the itch and the scratching impulse hit their peak and then gradually ease off. It's like a roller-coaster—unpleasant and compelling. As it eased off, I grab some lotion and run it onto my arm, and that helps—like I was being really caring to myself in a whole new way. I spend my days caring for others, and here I am learning to care for myself, ironic really (smiling)*

Every mindfulness practice can cultivate these foundational attitudes. Any mindfulness practice involves showing an interest in the climate of your mind and body. As you practice, try bringing an attitude of friendliness. You are learning to imbue your awareness with all the attitudes of practice, starting with interest, friendliness, appreciation, and care.

Attitudes can also be cultivated by practices tailored to develop these attitudes (you can listen to recordings at our website). The

> Each time you become aware of something pleasant is an opportunity to cultivate appreciation. Each time you become aware of something unpleasant is an opportunity to cultivate care.

following practice cultivates friendliness and compassion. It can help you recognize and work with reactivity. It can build your capacity for good will, toward yourself and others.

PRACTICE: Befriending Our Bodies and Minds

You can follow along on our website.

This practice starts in the usual way with choosing a stable posture, then gathering and anchoring your awareness. Then you go through a series of steps to cultivate friendliness. First see if you can be interested in whatever's happening in your body-mind, meeting it with kindness and care, even when it is unpleasant and painful. It can be helpful to cultivate a sense of well-wishing to use some phrases, under your breath, such as "Safe and well," "Peaceful," "Ease and kindness." In the next step you bring to mind someone with whom you have a positive relationship, then someone who is having some difficulty in their life. Finally, you turn toward yourself, wishing yourself well. Each step is about cultivating a sense of friendliness.

Try this befriending practice daily for a period of days or weeks. Remember, this is cultivation, so let go of forcing anything; you can't force a seed to germinate or a plant to grow. Give it the right conditions and time and then see what happens.

Befriending Your Mind in Everyday Life

Each day is a chance to cultivate these attitudes of mind. The everyday exercises and practices I'll introduce are just that, practicing a skill in your life so that it becomes a part of your life.

MOHAMMED: *I used to find my kids' relentless questions maddening. "Daddy, what's this, how many colors are in a rainbow, can a bird fly backwards, can I have an ice cream, will you push me on the swings?" I've started trying to see my kids not as maddening, but as teachers, in the sense that their curiosity has an innocence, freshness, and positive energy. They see the world and want to learn about it. That's a quality I'd like to have in my life. Yes, sometimes it is maddening; it's easier not to be curious, but it is worth it.*

LING: *I am scared of pain, physical and emotional pain. Scared it will trigger me or overwhelm me. I started small, with small moments that don't trigger me, but where I can practice being curious and kind. For example, if I feel bored, I instinctively reach for my phone or get busy. But when I am curious about boredom, it isn't so bad, and it can be interesting to lift the veil and ask, "What is this?" I moved on to spicy food, which I had always said I didn't like. But I realized that is something I do, blanket a whole set of experiences with "I don't like it." When I got curious, I realized good spicy food is interesting. I have started cooking some Thai curries, using green chiles, and moderating the spiciness with coconut milk. What a mixture that is. I love mixing up the two tastes and seeing the different results.*

As Mohammed and Ling describe, not only every day, but potentially any moment of our waking life is a chance to develop these attitudes and skills. There are also some tailored practices you can use in your everyday life.

EXERCISE: | **Acts of Kindness**

You can follow along on our website.

This practice cultivates kindness and generosity through action. It also lifts the spirits of those around us. Try committing to a few kind and generous acts each day. Perhaps start with just one a day and see how that goes. The kindness doesn't need to be a grand gesture; it can be as simple as greeting people with a smile, complimenting someone, or thanking someone who might not expect a thank you. Maybe you already do this. If you do, see if you can embody the kindness by practicing 50–50 awareness, keeping part of your awareness on the state of your body and mind before, during, and after the kind action. This connection to your body, emotions, and thoughts can help you register the impact of kindness. On some days, experiment with acts of kindness that are selfless. For example, doing something for someone without their knowledge, perhaps washing up a colleague's cup at work, leaving a sandwich for someone who is homeless and sleeping on the streets, leaving small gifts for people whose work you appreciate—paramedics, railway station staff, teachers, or the people who serve us in various places, supermarkets, restaurants, taxi drivers, or leave public restrooms as you would like to find them.

LING: *I picked up my daughter from the train station, and she was really upset because she had left her backpack on the train. "My phone and all my homework are in the bag," she wailed. It was late at night, and the station staff was getting ready to go home. But one of them said, "Don't worry. I'll phone the train manager and have them pass it to a train coming back this way. He made the call and said to take a seat on Platform 3 and wait for the train that will pull in at 11:23 P.M. and the train manager would have the bag. While we waited, we bought a large box of chocolates and left it for the station staff with a thank you note. "Thank you for going above and beyond and helping my daughter get her bag back." What is so interesting is that every time I go into the station now and see the staff working in this bustling station I have a sense of good will—even if the train is a bit late!*

The Ancient Oak and the Barefoot Professor:
Kindness in Action

The Barefoot Professor: An interesting research finding is how disconnected compassion for ourselves and others can be. What I mean is that people can be highly self-critical, but compassionate toward others.

The Ancient Oak: While this may be possible for a while, it is a recipe for burnout because in a way, kindness for ourselves and for others is the same thing. Being curious, friendly, and caring is an attitude of mind that cannot be reserved only for others or ourselves—it is in its essence the same; one cannot be truly, fully present without the other. So, we have to practice kindness for ourselves to be kind to others, and practice kindness for others to learn to be kind to ourselves.

The Barefoot Professor: This isn't easy because it can create harsh self-judgment for some people. So it's important, if we ask ourselves, "Why can I be kind to my children and speak so harshly to myself? That we do so with friendly curiosity. It is vital work, improving our sense of self-efficacy, creativity, and well-being. It turns out that being kind to others is good for us. These are not, as they're sometimes called, "random acts of kindness." As Sheila Gill, who teaches mindfulness for life, pointed out, it's not random at all; it's intentional—these are choices and actions intended to seed good.

EXERCISE: **Exploring Generosity**

You can follow along on our website.

Open both hands and imagine your left hand is holding an object you really value and cherish. What's it like to hold this thing that you cherish? Close your fingers around it so it is held protectively. Now have your open right hand ask your left, "Is that a gift for me? Can you share that with me?"
   What comes up for you?

You may find in this exercise that you value this object, but without a sense of grasping; your hand is ready to open like a bud in spring. Or you may covet it; our hand is like a steel fist. The request to share can elicit a wish to connect, wanting to share, protectiveness, resentment, or even anger. There is no right or wrong in this exercise; it is simply a way of playfully exploring how you relate to what you value, about protectiveness, about receiving and giving.

Befriending Your Mind
with Six Other Attitudes

Friends can come and go, but our minds are with us throughout our lives. That's a very good reason to befriend and take good care of your mind. It's also very helpful to become familiar with the six other attitudinal qualities that make your mind a good lifelong friend: patience, letting go, courage, trust, effort, and equanimity.

Patience

Impatience is understandable. We want what we want, *now*. We want what we don't want to go away, *now*. But being in a rush takes us out of this moment because we're trying to get somewhere else. An attitude of patience allows things to unfold in their own time.

> SOPHIA: *When my son was a young adult, he made what I regarded as some bad choices. I remember at one point he was besotted with this girl, and I was sure she was bad news. I wanted to do everything I could to help him see what I could see. If I am honest, I wanted to break up the relationship. So, I used the befriending practice, bringing his and my suffering to mind and trying to create a sense of good will and care, for him and for me. It dawned on me that she wasn't "bad news," but more of a "troubled soul." This helped me see that I had to step back, do nothing, be kind, and then* <u>*be patient*</u> *while everything ran its natural course. It took a year, and while it wasn't easy, by stepping back and being patient, I was able to see my tendency to want to fix everything. You can take the Sophia out of teaching, but you can't take the teacher out of Sophia!*

Patience works at different levels. At the most immediate and everyday level, you must be patient, waiting for the kettle to boil, someone to respond to an online inquiry, or for the traffic congestion to clear. At a deeper level, there are many parts of your life that take time—developing trust in a relationship, learning a new skill, and so on. Then at another level yet, much of what you really value takes patience because it takes time to evolve and develop: the development of deep love, real expertise, aging gracefully. In each of these areas, again, it's like gardening. You do the work of sowing seeds, tending the plants, but then step back and let them grow in their own time and way.

Patience makes it possible to enjoy tending the garden and in time enjoying the fruits of your work—greater focus, perspective, and the ability to speak and act wisely.

Letting Go

When we look inward, we soon notice how the mind wants to hold on to what we like and reject what we don't like. It's natural and compelling. This attitude of letting go means first seeing these tendencies, allowing them to be, and moving on—not clinging. Letting go can refer to our inner lives in terms of fixed ideas, habits, and stories that don't serve us. And it can refer to our outer lives, in terms of people, places, and things that similarly are no longer good for us or for them.

> ### The Ancient Oak: Letting Go
>
> Robert Pirsig in his book *Zen and the Art of Motorcycle Maintenance* describes how you can catch a monkey by tying a hollowed-out coconut to a stake in the ground and placing a banana so that the monkey must put its hand through the coconut shell to reach it. But once it grasps the banana, its fist is too large to pull back through the shell. Because it refuses to let go of the banana, you can catch the monkey.
>
> Sometimes when we grasp something, not letting go costs us; in the monkey's case it cost it its freedom and possibly its life.

SAM: *When my relationship broke up, it was my first heartbreak—he was my first love. Letting go of him was one thing, but I also had to let go of my idea of him and, in time, my grief too, so I could move forward. Sad tunes became my soundtrack, but it was all part of the letting go and moving forward with my life.*

What are the habits you hold on to in your life that don't serve you well? Are there areas where you find yourself striving, but it doesn't help, perhaps even sabotage you and create frustration? Overcommitting and then under-delivering, trying to change someone who never asked for your help, eating addictive food that you know is bad for you, excessive screen time, drinking too much alcohol, smoking? Is there a voice or pattern of self-talk that you allow, that is unfriendly—constantly criticizing, striving, making unhelpful comparisons, seeing yourself, other people, the world as not good enough? How would it be for you, like the monkey letting go of the banana, to let go of these habits and thoughts when you notice they don't serve you?

Courage

It takes courage to stop and look at ourselves and our lives and ask, "Am I living well? Am I living the life I imagined, the life I want to live?" It requires a certain willingness and openness to things we may prefer to avoid or run away from. To break out of habits, routines, and well-known identities and relationships takes courage. To turn toward difficult mind and body states like fear, anger, and disgust takes courage. The word *courage* in certain languages includes a sense of heart, which is perhaps why we've coined terms in English like "lionheart" and "brave heart."

> There is a "lionheartedness" in showing up, embracing life, making changes, and taking risks.

SAM: *When my first serious boyfriend ended our relationship, it felt like my heart—no, my whole life—got shattered into a million pieces. I just wanted to disappear, you know. It took a lot of courage to show up at work and face my friends. I was seriously scared I'd never be able to open up my heart again. But then, I took a walk with my mom, and we had this heart-to-heart like we never had before. She talked about her first love and how she managed to love again, my dad. They've been married 25 years now.*

Where in your life might this sense of lionheartedness be helpful? Speaking up, expressing feelings, including vulnerability and strength, navigating conflict, confronting fears that limit your life, taking risks personally and professionally that might enlarge your life, standing up for what you value and doing what you know is right and makes a difference.

Trust

Trust is the capacity to explore and respond to whatever life throws at us, both the small, day-to-day challenges and the inevitable larger challenges you'll face. What you're learning in mindfulness practice is an attitude of listening to your intuitions and beginning to honor and trust your experience. Inevitably, you will have doubts. Trust is being able to access a sense that you have what it takes to respond to challenges. You acknowledge the doubts, but you don't have to make them any larger than they need to be. Over time trust can develop a stable, enduring, unwavering quality. Seafarers take great care to ensure their boats are well built and maintained. They take them out to sea, where the conditions can easily turn very challenging, with confidence in the boat's seaworthiness. The ocean floor is littered with ships that have not weathered storms.

LING: *When a friend told me she'd seen my husband on a hookup app, I remember being overwhelmed with a sense of disbelief, hurt, anger: "That's it; that is a betrayal I can't get past." But then fear crept in as I realized I was dependent on him for money. Then there were the kids; they were still very little, and he was their dad. What would I do? How would I cope? It was a leap of faith, and I am not going to lie, I was really scared. I used my anger about his infidelity to help me take the leap. Somehow, I had a seed of courage deep inside me, fueled by anger, that I knew could grow into something. I had no idea what would happen, but deep down I trusted this barely discernible whisper of "Ling, you've got this."*

This sense of trust is something that emerges as you integrate mindfulness into your life. Where in your life do you have this sense of "I've got this?" When you've faced down fears and it worked out, in skills you've mastered over time, uncertainty you know you can ride out? Where can it be cultivated? Trust in yourself when you feel vulnerable, when you're recovering from an illness, that you can learn from setbacks. Trust in others—that good communication, boundaries, consistency, accountability, and reliability develop strong relationships in families, friendships, workplaces, and communities? Trust in the future, that if you individually and we collectively take care of one another and the planet, we will flourish?

Effort

We're used to hearing messages like "Make more of an effort," "Don't be lazy," "Hit the ground running," and "The only place success comes before work is in the dictionary," These messages are full of striving and harsh judgment. In the work of cultivating the mind, effort doesn't work the same way. Instead, effort is more like tuning a guitar string. If the guitar string is too tight, it twangs. If it is too loose, it lollops; both ways it's out of tune. Tuning a guitar involves getting it just right, not too tight, not too loose. Bringing mindfulness into your life is the same. Cultivating your mind requires an intentional and sustained effort—friendships don't happen by themselves. But striving is not always helpful. In fact, it can backfire.

MOHAMMED: *When I first started mindfulness practice, I thought it was like sports. If I trained hard, I would make gains. But I found myself getting really uptight—not just my mind but my body too, with thoughts like "You're a lousy meditator. Why can't you get this right?" This just made me even more uptight. I got curious and could see what the striving was doing to me, winding me up really tight. I have started to befriend my striving. Sometimes it serves me, like training in my home gym. But in many areas of life it doesn't, like when my back pain flares up.*

You're making a commitment to learning and growth, but as I keep reminding you, it's "cultivating the mind." Once you've done the work of planting the seeds and creating the right conditions, you're also letting it happen organically, without prodding and poking the soil and the seedling. This involves a subtle shift in which we care that we grow without trying to be "the best" at everything. It's an interesting practice to bring friendly interest to the question of what degree of effort is needed right now, both in your mindfulness practice and in your life.

Equanimity

We often waste a lot of energy refusing to accept things as they are, struggling to change things we don't want or like. Equanimity means learning to be with each moment as it is with a cool head and warm heart. This doesn't mean that you must like or accept everything about yourself and the world. Rather it is a poise and steadiness in the midst of your experience, the good and the bad. The art of balance and equanimity is something we'll explore in depth in Chapter 10.

Awareness becomes mindfulness when it is infused with all these attitudes. The awareness brings your life into focus, and the attitudes give it shape, color, and direction. But more than this, together they broaden horizons and build a sense of confidence and possibility.

Putting It All Together: A Mixing Board for the Mind

Sound engineers use mixing boards, where each channel can be dialed up and down. It is possible to think of all these attitudes of mindfulness in the same way as channels in a mixing board that you can choose to dial up or down, depending on the circumstances.

What does this mean in real life? We've all had the experience of not fully listening to someone, and what I am suggesting is that you can choose in any moment to dial your curiosity up and down, all the way from disinterest to awe.

SOPHIA: *In the final years of my mother's life, she suffered from dementia. She would often tell the same stories over and over again. I would find it upsetting. Sometimes I'd get irritated and lose my temper and be quite short with her. There was this one nurse in the residential home where my mother spent the last few months of her life who I learned a lot from. She would listen to my mother, but what she was really interested in was what was behind my mother's stories. Was she scared and needing reassurance, agitated, and needing help to calm down, or tired and needing to rest? In a sense she was dialing up her interest in what my mother was feeling and needing by listening to what she was communicating indirectly and nonverbally. I went home that night and realized the same is true in so many of my relationships.*

What Sophia is describing is learning from this nurse that she can reorient her attention from the stories themselves, which she's heard many times, to what her mother is saying nonverbally. And that here an interest, imbued with kindness and care, can help her come alongside her mother again. Of course, your level of interest depends in part on what you're paying attention to; some things are inherently more interesting than others. But what I am suggesting is you have choices about how much you infuse your attention with curiosity.

SOPHIA: *I remember my first day of school. I was petrified. I remember my mother saying, "Sophia, today is a day to put on your big girl pants." That encouragement to be brave meant a lot to me, and it's a phrase that's stuck with me throughout my life, a way to remind myself when I need to be courageous. Sometimes when I was a teacher and had a tricky day at work, on the way into work I'd say to myself, "Today is a day for my big girl pants."*

This is an example of Sophia's courage and knowledge that she can dial it up if she needs to. But mixing boards can do more than just dial channels up and down; they can be combined to create countless different effects. Sound engineers do this in music studios to produce different sounds. They can even simulate a small room, a large stadium, or a techno dance club. In the same way, you can mix these attitudes to create different states of mind. For example, for Sophia to communicate with her mother with dementia she needed to dial up interest in what her mother was communicating nonverbally, acceptance of the dementia diagnosis, letting go of how she wanted things to be, and a lot of patience. This creates the conditions for something different to happen in both the way Sophia feels about her mother and how she can be with her mother.

This is lifelong learning. You can try out what it is like to dial different attitudes up and down, in your mindfulness practice and everyday life. If you can do this while watching for what does and doesn't work for you, you can learn what each situation needs. In the same way that attention can be retrained, over time if you persist, it becomes second nature to know when and how to deploy them.

Cultivating the Ten Attitudes of Mind in Real Life, for Life

All the mindfulness practices you've learned so far can be elaborated by building these attitudes into your practice.

Mindfulness Practices

This might mean starting a practice by saying to yourself, for example, "I am committing this practice to developing my ability to let go." Then throughout the practice each time an opportunity presents itself to practice this attitude, you can work with it. For example, a problem in the day ahead might create a "monkey fist" in your mind. This is a chance to let go, maybe saying something under your breath to support your letting go of these states of mind—"let go of the banana." Finally, at the end of the practice you might form an intention to check in throughout the day if there is a need or chance to practice whatever attitude you're looking to cultivate. For example, "Each time I find myself getting caught up in worry today, I'll practice letting go of the banana."

You can also play with the idea of the mixing board. During a practice, you might ask, "What does this moment need?" This could mean what attitudes, dialed up to what degree, in what combination will serve me here? This is not a problem to be solved intellectually or something to get right or be good at. Instead, returning to the word *cultivation*, it is more of a question of what combination of conditions will cultivate the garden of your mind. This can be creative. Choose which attitudes or combination of attitudes you'd like to cultivate. Choose language that resonates for you. Finally, set up the practice in whatever way supports you best.

LING: *When I was first separated from my husband, my confidence was rock bottom, and I was really scared. I was in therapy, and my therapist helped me rebuild my self-confidence and life. I remember putting up a picture board near where I meditate with a picture of my therapist and my best friends so I could see them. I'd start my practice by looking at the board, which reminded me I have love and support. Then during the practice, after I'd settled my mind, I used this phrase, which somehow really spoke to me "May I be open-hearted and lionhearted." I ended the practice by bringing to mind the parts of the day I needed to be open-hearted and the parts of the day I needed to be lionhearted and made a commitment to be those things in those moments. I did this for a few months, and it helped me go into each day with a sense that I could meet the day and be kind, caring, and courageous.*

SOPHIA: *When I knew I would be seeing my son with his girlfriend, I would use my mindfulness practice to prepare myself beforehand. I'd start the practice with an intention to develop my ability to be kind, let go and be patient. There was lots of grist for the mill, as I knew I would find it hard to see them together, to see them gaslighting each other. As I was sitting meditating, I was very aware that I wanted to intervene. So, I'd say under my breath, tongue in cheek, "letting go of the banana." I'd have a sense of my mind like a fist opening and letting go of my fixation on doing something. At the end of the practice, I would bring them to mind arriving for dinner and play the evening like a video, practicing at various trigger points being patient and letting go.*

There have long been practices in contemplative traditions to cultivate different attitudes of mind. Here are a few examples of phrases that are often used in these practices. The phrases often start with something like, "May I be . . ." or "May you be." Then you can add different words depending on what it is you're cultivating.

> To cultivate appreciation: Happy and easily contented; Live with ease and joy. Open to loving and being loved; Take joy in good fortune. May ease and contentment continue; Grateful for all that I have in my life
>
> To cultivate kindness: Live with ease and kindness
>
> To cultivate compassion: Safe and protected; Free from suffering and the causes of suffering; Find peace in the midst of this
>
> To cultivate courage: Capable and dignified; Live lightly; Lionhearted: Be brave even when I am afraid
>
> To cultivate letting go: Live lightly; Put down unhelpful thoughts and habits; Let go of the past; Let go of thinking.
>
> To cultivate equanimity: Balanced and centered; Allow things to be as they are; Finding peace amid all life's changes and challenges; Steady; Nothing to change, nothing to fix

Only do what is helpful. So, with these phrases, that means learning what is needed in any particular moment and returning to the idea of the mixing board, perhaps combining the cultivation of attitudes together, as we saw with Ling: "May I be open-hearted and lionhearted." Finally, this is about befriending your mind so you can live in the world, so you can use these phrases in relation to yourself, other people, or the wider world. You can follow some of these practices on our website.

SOPHIA: *When I was a teacher, we had this new principal at my school, and she made a lot of changes, which was unsettling for everyone. In that period my daily mindfulness practice included the phrases "May I be safe and open-minded, may all the people I encounter today be safe and happy, and may my school be a place of safety and playful learning." I'd sometimes return to these phrases in moments throughout the day. I found it affected how I was throughout the day, and not only helped me stay steady through the changes but also create a sanctuary in my classroom for the children. The changes were unsettling, yes, but necessary, and I went on to head up a department in the school with the principal, and that school became a school the children took real pride in.*

Everyday Life and the Wider World

Befriending your mind on its own doesn't necessarily change anything in your life. But what it can do is create the conditions for you to respond differently. Difficulties become less threatening, and you have more of a sense of confidence that you can work with them. You come to recognize the many good moments in your day, see them more clearly, and understand what they have to offer us. This is where change happens in your life because it translates to what you say and do, and over time this shapes your relationships and life.

The Ancient Oak and the Barefoot Professor:
The Rūmī "Guest House" Poem Again

The Ancient Oak: In Rūmī's "Guest House" poem, he encourages us to recognize and welcome "a joy, a depression, a meanness" because we can learn from them all. Curiosity and friendliness help us open the door and greet these guests, appreciation helps us savor the joy, and care helps us respond to the depression. So the attitudes support us in becoming a friend to our inner world.

The Barefoot Professor: Barbara Fredrickson is a professor of psychology at the University of North Carolina at Chapel Hill and has developed the broaden-and-build theory. Her work has shown that positive attitudes like curiosity broaden and build our attention and sense of self-efficacy. They widen and brighten the lens of our flashlight of awareness and then make us feel like we cope better.

The Ancient Oak and the Barefoot Professor: So, what we're saying is that these attitudes support us to recognize and welcome the positive and negative in both our inner landscape (a passing thought or a feeling of love for a friend) and our outer world (a brief encounter with someone during our day, birth of a child, retirement). We see the world more clearly, as having more possibilities, and ourselves as more resilient.

The people we're around and the places we spend time in not only affect our mood but can also shape who we are. One of the most important ways for you to cultivate these attitudes is to find people and places that embody the very attitudes you'd like to cultivate. You have choices about how, with whom, and where you spend your time. So, make these choices intentionally and wisely. Of course, this isn't always completely possible, but it is rarely all or nothing. Perhaps you can't choose where you work, but you can make some adjustments.

> Friendship isn't always easy, we don't always like everything about our friends, and friendships can ebb and flow. But a good friendship is one in which we can see and be seen, including the light, dark, and shadow and through different seasons of our life.

SAM: *Working in the health service isn't a ride in the park. Cynicism and burnout are like the climate. But you know what? I really love the patient work, and I'm all in. If I spend time with colleagues who are cynical, it rubs off on me. So I have mastered the art of dodging my most cynical colleagues during breaks. And if I can't, I try to steer what we talk about to something positive. It's not just the climate in my head; it's the whole scene I'm in.*

You are shaped by and shape your world. This wider context for mindfulness is something I'll return to in Chapters 11 and 12.

TROUBLESHOOTING: Befriending Your Body–Mind Can Throw Up Blocks and Obstacles

Self-Judgments and "Backdraft." It's not uncommon for befriending to trigger a tirade of unhelpful thoughts, such as "I don't deserve this," "Other people are better than me," "Lay low, tall poppies get scythed down," "This is woo woo nonsense," "Toughen up and get on with it," "This is self-indulgent," "I have to get this right," or even "I can't do this; it's too hard for me." These thoughts require the very attitudes I've set out in this chapter, such as curiosity, kindness, care, trust, and letting go. When they come up, ask yourself, "Which attitudes might serve me well?" It's hard to be genuinely curious, kind, and caring at the same time as being judgmental. The mindfulness practices are a chance to practice listening with friendly and caring interest for our own reactivity, including the voice in our head that reacts to the invitation to befriend our minds with judgments.

In extreme cases there can even be backdraft. *Backdraft* refers to opening the door to a room where there is a fire, and the sudden influx of oxygen feeds the fire, in extreme cases even creating a fireball. The same can be true for people prone to very negative thinking, for whom friendliness oxygenates the self-criticism, in extreme cases even creating a sense of "I am unlovable." It is important to tailor these practices so that they work for you and for where you are just now in your life. The befriending practice and kindness can come to be straightforward at a stable and steady time in our lives. But at times when you're busy or stressed you may need something else: rest or the support of a good friend for example.

Parts of us that feel, or sometimes are excluded, different, marginalized, or hard to reach. The way you feel and are treated in the world will likely be mirrored in your practice. You may have habits, parts of your personality, or even attributes that elicit guilt or shame or that others find hard to accept or perhaps actively discriminate against. This might be your sex, gender, skin color, weight, sexuality, or things you've done that either you're not proud of and/or others disapprove of. What can happen is you hide or turn away from these parts of yourself. In your mindfulness practice, see if you can include, even welcome, these different parts of yourself, those that want to be here, those that don't, that feel included, feel excluded, feel okay, feel not okay, that you'd like to see the light of day but keep hidden in the shadows.

"I can be generous to others, but not to myself." As with compassion, real, deep generosity is something that flows through us, regardless of whether it is directed at ourselves or others. Having a genuinely healthy relationship with others requires a healthy relationship with ourselves. So, developing these attitudes toward yourself is an investment in your capacity to extend them to others.

Sometimes trying to approach things in a new way triggers zoning out. This might simply be the mind wandering. Or it can be a way of the mind saying, "No, I'm not doing this." The way to work with zoning out is first to recognize it and then to allow these reactions—they are all part of the mind's natural reactivity. The first time you try to stand back from and see yourself zoning out can be quite difficult and a little strange. Befriending is learning to care deeply about both yourself and others and then choosing an appropriate response.

Feeling hopeless about change. Our prevailing attitudes can be deeply ingrained, and it is easy to get exasperated or start despairing. But everything, including this reactivity—"I can't do this; it's who I am"—is grist for the mill. Approach it as best you can with a renewed curiosity, friendliness, and care. Like all capacities, when you work on them, especially in the face of real difficulty, they grow. Persistence, with these attitudes, builds a sense of self-confidence and can open the possibility of the most rewarding and perhaps most difficult work. Rather than turn away in fear or judgment, or feel overwhelmed, you can recognize and welcome them; perhaps they have come to teach you something.

There are also *powerful prevailing cultural attitudes*, so what we're doing is in a sense more than simply obstacles in the mind; it is countercultural. I have described a healthy mind as one that can be kind and caring, but in some contexts kindness and compassion are seen as weak. I have described a healthy mind as one that calibrates effort, is patient, and knows when to let go, but striving is often highly valued in workplaces, schools, and families. Finally, I have described a healthy mind as one that is capable of appreciation, but some people might describe appreciation as indulgence: a scathing voice that says, "You think a lot of yourself." Awareness enables you to really see when these ideas come up and how they affect your mind and your life. This spirit of inquiry is at the heart of mindfulness for life, so you can learn from your experience what serves you and what doesn't.

We've seen how Sam, Mohammed, Ling, and Sophia cultivated these attitudes to create connection, as an antidote to striving, to dismantle an inner critic and make important life changes. Dolly Parton is incredibly successful both in her art and in business. Here is how she resolved this question of keeping an open heart for her art while having strength as a businesswoman. "As a writer, I have to leave my heart open. . . . Because as a writer, if you harden your heart, you're not going to feel all that emotion you need to feel, and you won't be able to write what people feel." She then explains that to be a businesswoman, she learned *to strengthen the muscles around her heart.*

Being Your Own Lifelong Friend

Steadying and anchoring awareness was only the first part of the story. The attitudes you bring to awareness are the next part of the story. When awareness is infused with these attitudes, it is illuminated. When this is aligned with your values, it can shape the direction of your life. This is what we turn to in the chapters ahead.

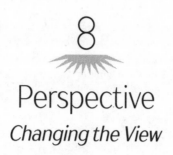

8

Perspective
Changing the View

Sophia, waking at 3:21 A.M.: Oh no, I really needed a good night's sleep.
I feel wide awake. I may as well check my phone. There are messages
from both my kids . . . they've had an argument. Oh no, is it my fault?
Did I do something wrong? Maybe like me and my sister they're always
going to have a difficult relationship. . . . There is that numbness in
my fingers again; I've been putting off seeing my doctor. I hope it's
nothing. . . . The tap in the bathroom is dripping; I need to get that
fixed. . . . Why can't I sleep? I'm going to be tired tomorrow.

Like Sophia, we've all awakened in the middle of the night. The dark, soli-
tude, and quiet provide just the right conditions for this sort of rumination
and worry. You've learned to gather and anchor your attention and to start the
process of befriending your body–mind. This helps us begin to see sensations
as sensations, moods as moods, impulses as impulses, thoughts as thoughts.
Rather than be carried away by your thoughts and feelings, you can stay steady
and see what is happening. This is the first step in being able to stand back and
take a different perspective, the focus of this chapter.

> **The Barefoot Professor and the Ancient Oak: Perspective**
>
> **The Barefoot Professor:** Human beings evolved with this capacity to think
> and reflect on what is happening. It is arguably something that is unique to
> our species, at least in as much as we also use language to describe what we see.
> We're not born with this capacity; it develops in childhood and adolescence.
> Infants simply are contented, hungry, cold. In the first weeks and months of
> life, they can't even distinguish their experience from other people's. A loud

sound is simply experienced as alarming, a caregiver's fearful face is fear. Only some way into infancy do we learn to separate ourselves from others, and only later in childhood do we learn to see other people's points of view.

The Ancient Oak: I don't want to tread on your toes. I know Einstein was a scientist like you, but he was also someone who thought about his scientific work in a much broader context. He wrote, "The true value of a human being is determined primarily by the measure and the sense in which he has attained to liberation from the self." He is pointing to the tremendous value of being able to step out of our narrow and limited personal perspective.

A Different Point of View

There are several ways our perspective changes. Here are some of the main ones.

Grounding

The simplest and most direct way to shift out of worry, restlessness, and reactivity is to ground yourself in your body. This is the idea of "coming home to our bodies" discussed in Chapter 3. Your body is always with you, and there is always somewhere in your body that you can anchor. Grounding is an intentional shift into awareness of the body, which of course shifts us out of our heads.

> SOPHIA: *I've learned that disappearing into a vortex of worry in the middle of the night is a surefire way to not get back to sleep. So I went to the bathroom, drank some water, and when I got back into bed, I got comfortable on my back, did a Breathing Space, and then started body scanning, taking lots of time in my toes and feet, knowing that they were a long way away from my head. When the worries came back, I said to the worries, "I see you; I'll deal with you tomorrow." They kept coming back, so I went downstairs and wrote them down on my to-do list for tomorrow, and said, "Right, worries, you stay down here; see you tomorrow." I went back to bed and to the body scanning. This time I must have fallen asleep before I got to my torso.*

Grounding awareness in our bodies takes us out of our heads and breaks the chains of reactivity. Instead of worry developing into generalized anxiety, it becomes a temporary flurry of worry that we have recognized and chosen not to allow to escalate. Instead of rumination developing into feeling low, even depressed, it becomes more like some dark clouds passing through.

Zooming In and Zooming Out

Mindfulness practices teach you that you can zoom in and zoom out, just like you can with a flashlight or a camera. For example, in a Body Scan you can come as close as is okay to sensations and then step back again to see the sensations moment by moment. You can zoom right out and see the whole body floodlit in awareness, open to the myriad sensations in any given moment.

> SAM: *My father was an engineer whose work took him to different countries. Until I was nine, we traveled with him. He was working in Botswana, and we lived in this bungalow surrounded by cool tropical trees. Whenever life got too much, I'd climb one of the trees without telling anyone and hang out there. Picture this: me on a branch stretching over the driveway, feeling like I'm straight outta Jungle Book, rolling with Mowgli and Bagheera. From that treetop spot, I'd scope out everything—people coming and going, my dog doing his thing, and my family doing what they do. It was like my secret sanctuary, this perch where I could check out the world from a whole new angle.*

> SOPHIA: *The thoughts at 3:00 A.M.—"My kids' argument is my fault; the numbness in my fingers might be something serious; I am going to be tired tomorrow"—are like sitting at a railroad crossing in my car, watching a freight train with dozens of cars thundering by, each with these worry thoughts written on the side. It can be scary and overwhelming. Taking a Breathing Space is like driving up to the hills above the railway crossing, parking, and looking down the hill at the vista. The train is still there, down the hill, moving through the countryside, I can still make out the words on the sides of the cars; they're smaller but still readable. But now the scene in front of me includes other parts of my life, my friends, my boyfriend, my grandchild, Noah. I can even, if I try to, get the sense of all the people whose lives I've touched in my teaching career.*

Stepping Back

Stepping back is zooming out to the next level. It involves taking a step backward to see all that is happening from a wider perspective. Psychologists call this "perspective broadening." It pulls us out of reactivity and helps us see more clearly. Putting something into perspective often creates a sense that this is something you can handle.

> SAM: *Nursing, especially in intensive care, is no joke. All high stakes, equipment galore, zero outside windows, sick patients, and a bunch of stressed-out relatives. It's intense! So when I catch a break I make a beeline outside and, if I have time, hike up to this bench on the hillside where I can kick back with a coffee and a snack and take in the view. From up there I can see the hospital, but also the downtown, where I go out with*

friends. I can see one of my biking routes snaking along the river, cutting through the park and out of town. It's like my escape route to sanity, you know? Getting out of the hospital bubble for a bit and putting things into perspective.

LING: *Sometimes I get consumed by thoughts like "I am a not a good person" and "I am unlovable." They are like wrecking ball thoughts; they knock me flying. It's taken me some time, and calling them "wrecking ball thoughts" was part of the process. It helped me realize I can step back and rather than be crushed by these thoughts I can watch them swing through like a wrecking ball. When I do this, they lose their destructive power.*

Time Travel

We have this extraordinary capacity to remember, to plan, and to forecast. Regret is an example of time travel back in time that can cause us pain. Worry is an example forward in time that causes anxiety. Regret, worry, rumination, and fantasy are rarely intentional; more likely, they capture our attention and take us away from this moment. But you can also use time travel intentionally to shift perspective in ways that are helpful.

MOHAMMED: *My elder daughter has always been a worrier. What most kids will brush off she tends to hang on to and worry about: "We're going to be late! Have we forgotten the soccer cleats? Why was I not invited to Melissa's birthday party?" So, we got this big jar, and we labeled it the "Worry Jar." I got her to write her worries down on a piece of paper and put them in the jar, and she tries to let them go as she puts them into the jar. That was only a bit helpful, but what has proved much more helpful is going back to the jar and picking out the worries a few weeks or even months later. Normally she laughs and says, "My goodness, I can't believe I was worried about that—that's so silly."*

Worry is our mind creating stories about all the ways things might go wrong. The contents of worry are not that important; you can substitute any plotline. It works just as well for trivial and serious, imagined, and real issues. Our interconnectedness, social media, and 24/7 news means there is a ready supply of things to worry about. The worry jar is very good at teaching us that what can dominate our minds now is often not that serious later. The bigger lesson, especially for people prone to worry, is that anxiety isn't normally about the *content* of our worries but rather the *process* of latching on to something and then obsessively trying to solve it by thinking about it over and over.

You can play with time travel by choosing different places in time to stand.

LING: *I remember a moment negotiating my divorce, especially childcare, the family home, and money—things got very difficult. I found it hard to remember what it was like when we were first together, but I tried hard. We once loved each other; we had a lot of fun pre-kids. And when our kids were little, we were a good team. Then I thought forward to how I wanted us to be able to do things like birthdays, weddings, and funerals as a family. This helped me make compromises so we could get to something that worked best for our kids and for both of us. I made sure all we decided was fair, but my destination was making sure that should our kids get married, he and I could sit next to each other amicably at their wedding ceremonies.*

You can go backward or forward in minutes, days, years, or even a whole lifetime. You can imagine your 30-, 40-, 50-, 60-, 70-, or 80-year-old selves and ask, "What would they make of this moment?"

SOPHIA: *My will includes a statement of wishes. I have asked that my headstone include on it: "A life well-lived." I think about this sometimes, especially if I feel stuck. It reminds me that in the end that's what it is all about, living my life as best I can. This long view puts it all in perspective.*

Taking Someone Else's Point of View

We see the world through our own eyes. But in any scene, there are as many perspectives as there are people. It is natural of course that you see the world from your perspective, but you forget that is all it is, your perspective.

MOHAMMED: *One of my kids' favorite things to do is to go down to the river and feed the geese. There is a spot where a large flock of geese hang out. They recognize us, and when they see us, they come onto land and will eat out of our hands. The kids love it. Last Sunday morning we were feeding the geese when all a sudden all hell broke out. The kids were terrified by the sudden honking, hissing, and flapping as the geese took off, just as a large dog came running toward us, barking. I picked up my youngest child, and the older one grabbed my leg and hid behind me. Then the dog's owner, a woman laughing and talking on the phone, came around the corner. I heard her say to whoever she was talking to, "My dog just scared off like a hundred geese from the path. That will teach them; no one can have picnics here because the geese terrorize you begging for food."*

How you see the world is shaped by all that you've learned up until this moment. This example shows how the same situation was experienced differently by Mohammed, his children, and the dog owner. Mohammed feels scared, protective of his kids, and then angry about the dog. His kids liked the geese, but their sudden change into a honking, hissing, flapping flock scared them. The dog was big, off the lead, barking, and running toward them. Not surprisingly, they were also scared by the dog. The woman was amused and pleased her dog had chased away the geese. To her the geese were a nuisance that meant she hadn't been able to picnic at her local park. She was too busy talking to her friend on the phone to really notice Mohammed and his kids. Each experienced their own perspective as their reality. But without the ability to see others' viewpoints and change our viewpoint, we can easily misunderstand others, become fixed and dogmatic, and get into arguments with others who don't share our viewpoint.

> We see the world through the lens of all we've learned before.

Shifting perspective can include choosing to see through someone else's eyes. Friends sometimes ask one another for advice: "What do you think? What would you do?" Often, you can see a friend's problem quite clearly, because you're seeing it from the outside and you care about them. You can choose to ask yourself, "How would a friend see my situation, and what might they say?" Perhaps you have a friend who never judges you, another who is wise, and yet another who tells you straight up what you need to hear. You can choose these different friends' perspectives, depending on what you need. It can extend beyond this, to people you trust and respect—mentors, parents, grandparents, and so on. The intention is simple, to choose someone whose perspective might be helpful.

Shifting Modes of Mind

You've started to learn that you have these two modes of mind, experiencing this moment directly or thinking about what's happening. You've started to move between experiencing and thinking, with a sense of which is helpful to you in different situations and at different times. We explored this in Chapter 3. Stepping back and observing enables us to see the experiencing and thinking modes of mind and the movement between them.

MOHAMMED: *I have learned, mostly through the Body Scan and mindful movement, that I can notice the pain in my back and move up close to the unpleasant sensations. When I do this more often than not, they change—sometimes they get tighter or more spread out. Paying attention brings the sensations into the foreground, and that can feel intense. If I start to think about the pain, it tends to go to a bad place quite quickly: "This pain has been around so long. I am going to have to live with this for such a long time, and I am not sure I can—it's too much." I try to unhook from the word* pain, *especially* chronic pain. *This means I can see the sensations as something I can work with, and I can ask, "What do I need right now?" When I zoom out, I can also hold my whole body in awareness. When my whole body is floodlit, the unpleasant sensations sit alongside parts of my body that are doing just fine, and thoughts and feelings that are about stuff in my life other than the unpleasant sensations. I am not my pain. That is so important. I have met people in rehab who have become their chronic pain, and I get it, but that is not a good place.*

This observer mode helps us see what is happening more clearly, which in turn means you can choose what you pay attention to and how you pay attention. As the example above illustrates, it added to Mohammed's toolkit for working with pain.

Doing Nothing

Because inevitably things change, if you stand still, you can wait and watch the world around you change, as well as the landscape of your mind and body. Doing nothing can be counterintuitive but can also be just what is needed.

LING: *My kids when they were toddlers, like all toddlers, would have tantrums. But my daughter could get into a real state and have a lot of trouble getting out of it. We had this book we'd read called* Sometimes I'm Bombaloo *by Rachel Vail. It describes a child, Katy Honors, who has a brilliant way of describing what it's like to be in a funk: "scrunchy face," fist banging, foot stamping, pointing, yelling. She calls it bombaloo and describes beautifully why tantrums don't respond to reason: "When I'm bombaloo I don't want to think about it, I want to smash stuff." Bombaloo became a word we used in our family. It helped to give a name to this scary state toddlers can get into. Everyone understood if someone was bombaloo what that was like; that they needed time and love and that it would pass. In the book, in one scene Katy Honors throws her clothes around her room in a rage and ends up with some underpants on her head. This makes her laugh and breaks the bombaloo spell. It's a book that passed around to quite a few of our friends too.*

Of course, knowing when to do nothing and when to act requires experience and wisdom, and we'll get to that in later chapters. For now, you can note that by standing still you will inevitably see change, and sometimes, as with toddlers' tantrums, it is your only real choice. Doing nothing also shifts us out of the modes of doing and fixing, which is a change in and of itself.

Learning to Change Our Perspective

We have this extraordinary capacity to see one another's point of view, to step back and take a wider view, and to time travel. How can you develop this skill so you can use it intentionally in ways that serve you?

Mindfulness Practices

Again, all the mindfulness practices taught in this book will help you learn these skills. Every practice involves grounding and anchoring, learning to zoom in, zoom out, and observe all that is happening. Every practice involves switching between experiencing, thinking, and observing. In any given moment you can separate out all the components of your experience and see it for what it is, a coming together of body sensations, feelings, impulses, and thoughts; nothing more and nothing less. Zooming in and out helps you move in to explore and stand back to take a wider view. Finally, every practice involves seeing what happens when you step back and do nothing. Perspective taking is learned in all the mindfulness practices.

> SAM: *Dealing with psoriasis, my skin can get crazy itchy. At first, I was worried that mindfulness would mess with me because it made me pay attention to something I usually tried to brush off, the skin irritation. And yeah, paying attention? Just creates an overwhelming urge to scratch. But I realized that just tuning in isn't mindfulness. I figured out that it's also being curious, patient, and brave. When I added these attitudes to the mix, it was like I was holding the flashlight. And now the illumination was helpful. I could zero in on the part of my body that was doing fine, like my feet, then zoom out to other parts. Sometimes I throw in some music that I can tune in to. And a little self-discovery: I'm pretty darned impatient. Just naming that with a bit of kindness made me see the power of patience.*

The Breathing Space is a practice that you can use anywhere, any time, to help you step out of autopilot, note the landscape of your body and mind, gather and anchor your attention, and then in the third and final step broaden your awareness to your body and wider experience. (If you want to refresh your memory, see Chapter 3.) Like all the mindfulness practices, it can ground you and provide a wider perspective. In Step 3 of the Breathing Space you can involve any of the strategies above: grounding, zooming out, shifting perspective across time or to another person's viewpoint. Our mindfulness practice, like a good friend, is always there. It doesn't judge us; it cares and can help us.

Changing Perspective in Real Life, for Life

SOPHIA: *When my parents retired, they joined a university that offers courses for older adults. They did a course on the poet Rilke and were forever quoting him. I remember them saying they wanted to follow Rilke's advice and live their lives in ever-increasing circles. They did. My father worked as a postman into his 80s just so he could chat with people on his route, and my mother was part of the church, helping it with its outreach work.*

Taking It Further: Developing Your Ability to Change Perspective in Life, for a Lifetime

All the skills and practices I have introduced can be explored for a lifetime as you apply them to new and varied situations and scenarios that are more charged, complex, unknown, or uncertain. For example, anchoring is relatively easy when all is well, but when things get more challenging, you need to find a way to stay rooted, flexible, and strong while the weather system moves through.

> The ability to shift perspective can help us live our lives in ever-increasing circles. It gives us a fresh perspective on where we are in any moment; it enables us to imagine what is possible and to pick out a way of getting there.

The attitudes of mindfulness are your friend. What happens when you take a deliberate stance of interest, kindness, and care? Maybe revisit Chapter 7 and bring these attitudes into play here. You will more than likely find that as you become more familiar with your mind and body, and you are able to bring not only perspective, but perspective imbued with interest, kindness, and care, you will intuitively know which approach to take. And that with patience, persistence, and time this will become second nature.

This practice develops this sense of rootedness, strength, and steadiness so you can keep perspective through different conditions and circumstances. Instilling it with curiosity, appreciation, care, and trust enriches it.

PRACTICE: Tree

You can follow along on our website.

In the tree practice, you bring to mind a tree that you think of as being strong, vital, and flexible. Next, you imagine becoming the tree and lightly scan through your body, from the roots up through the trunk, through the branches, to the crown of your head, the top of the tree. Recognize what sensations are around, perhaps lightly naming them. End the scanning with a sense of your whole body, breathing like a tree.

Now, in the same way that a tree stays strong and flexible to moment-by-moment changes, see if you can respond to whatever comes up. Then, as you bring the practice to a close, form an intention to take this sense of rootedness, strength, and responsiveness into your day. There may be moments you can bring to mind from the day ahead where this might be particularly helpful, maybe play them through your mind, with this sense of yourself as rooted, strong, and flexible, like a tree.

This practice is intended to develop a sense of steadiness, balance, and strength from which you can view your life. Trees also get us through difficulties like a squall passing through, high winds, a dry summer, a hard winter. The comparison with a tree can help you relate to the inevitable disappointments, losses, and frustrations, as well as joys, pleasures, and moments of connection in your life.

The Barefoot Professor: Trees and Brain Networks

Trees are also a useful metaphor in understanding the brain. Professor Lisa Feldman-Barrett explains that our nervous system is made up of 128 billion individual neurons that are organized into networks. Each neuron looks like a tree, communicating with other trees through its branches (dendrites), trunks (axons), and roots. The communication between the neurons, like trees, is through chemicals. Like any ecosystem, our neurons are a huge interconnecting network. The brain develops in childhood through a process of tuning and pruning—what is used is tuned; what is less used is pruned.

There are many metaphors in nature with which you can explore perspective. You can imagine forests, lakes, rivers, estuaries, and mountains and use them as a way to see the changing conditions in your body, mind, and life. The changing weather and seasons can be like the changes in your body and mind. A squall can be like a powerful burst of energy. A sunny day can bring a sense of warmth, stillness, and contentment. A period of depression can be like a long winter. And wider than all of these, the sky can be like awareness that sits above and encompasses it all with extraordinary spaciousness.

Emily Dickinson reminds us in her poem "There Is Another Sky" that around the world everyone is experiencing both the same and a different sky:

And there is another sunshine, though it be darkness there. I am writing this in New Zealand, which is 12 hours ahead of where most of my family and friends live. As the sun rises here, in this moment, I know it is going down for them. Changing perspective is reminding yourself of all these different ways you can shift perspective.

SOPHIA: *I can relatively easily anchor in my breathing. If I am a little bit distracted, putting my hand on my belly helps. But I needed this tree practice and years of trial and error to develop ways of grounding myself in more difficult situations. When I am with people, becoming aware of my posture helps a lot. I bring to mind the tree standing strong and resolute. If there is a lot of emotion, to me this is like a lot of weather—wind gusts, rain, hail, and frost. Having a sense of my feet rooted in the ground helps. If I am really activated, my body is too stimulated, I stay with the idea of the tree, but now I pay attention to myself as part of a whole forest of trees standing together, providing protection to one another.*

Sophia's example shows her skillfully choosing to place her attention in different places depending on her state of mind and what is going on. This exploration and learning can be revisited in an ongoing way.

SAM: *I was best man at my friend Adam's wedding. I hate speaking in public. As the big day approached, I was all tangled up in anxiety, hot, my heart beating, and all these images of me blowing it. It was a freaking nightmare. I tried switching it up. Instead of its being about <u>my fear of blowing it</u>, I flipped the script. I made it about <u>doing right by Adam</u>. It was his day, you know. Suddenly it wasn't about me and my messing up anymore; he and his partner were what it was all about.*

We can zoom out, standing back to see the bigger picture.

MOHAMMED: *I remember once when I was playing college sports, we were traveling to a game through a rural area when we came to a tree that had fallen across the road. It was clear that it would take hours to clear, and there was no other route that would get us there in time. We'd been there about half an hour and were stressed out trying to figure out a solution when a minivan pulled up on the other side of the tree, the driver looking equally concerned. She was taking her visiting elderly parents back to the airport and would miss the flight if she had to backtrack to an alternative route. My father was good at solving problems, and he took a bird's-eye view of the situation and came up with an amazing solution: "How about we swap cars, you take mine and turn around to the airport and I take yours so Mohammed can make his game? We can exchange numbers and arrange later tonight to swap cars back on the way home again." That's what we did.*

PRACTICE: **Changing Perspective**

You can follow along on our website.

This changing perspective mindfulness practice uses all that you have learned to play with perspective. You start by stabilizing and grounding yourself and then broaden your awareness out to a sense of the whole body. Scan lightly through your body and notice the myriad sensations you feel. Then bring to mind something in your life that is an issue for you but a manageable one, and note any resonance in your body, your mood state, any thoughts, or images that come up.

Now, with a spirit of interest and playfulness, you can try different points of view. *Ground in your body*, choosing somewhere to anchor your awareness in this moment, and ask yourself what your experience of this issue is. *Now change your perspective in time* and see how the issue you chose looks from these different timepoints.

Finally, take someone else's point of view (or more than one) and ask yourself how the issue looks from these different people's points of view.

Letting go of these different perspectives, come back to your anchor and your body. What, if anything, can you take into your day going forward?

There is no right or wrong way to do this practice, nor is there something you're trying to achieve. Try to approach the practice in a spirit of exploration: "I wonder what I will discover?"

MOHAMMED: *I was so angry with the woman whose dog scared my kids. I was barely aware of it, but the anger gripped my body, especially my face, shoulders, and hands, and my back pain became a shooting pain up my spine. A red mist came over me, and my impulse was to pick up a stick and beat the dog and then shout at the owner. I am not proud of this, but it is what I felt. I didn't pick up a stick or shout. I stayed anchored in my hands. I stood and stretched out, and slowly the red mist cleared enough for me to try shifting into the dog and the owner's viewpoint. I even tried seeing it from the point of view of someone else walking by. We had a dog growing up. He loved being off the lead, chasing through woods and fields after squirrels and rabbits. The dog was doing what dogs love to do. Yes, she should have had control of her dog, but as far as I can tell she was not aware of me and my kids, and she wasn't trying to scare anyone. I guess the person walking by might see her perspective and mine equally. I resolved, with no hurry, to say hello to the dog next time I saw him, and if he is friendly, have my kids say hello so they don't become afraid of dogs. I suspect he is friendly; otherwise his owner wouldn't let him off the lead in a park where there are often kids.*

The perspective practice is intended to be used flexibly. At different times, different approaches will be called for—grounding, shifting time frame, seeing it from someone else's point of view. Each element can also be used flexibly, choosing where and how to anchor your awareness, which time frame, which person's perspective.

Enriching Your Ability to Change Perspectives in Different Situations

Much of our life centers around the family, friends, co-workers, and others who are part of our day-to-day lives. We're social animals, able to form attachments, manage hierarchies, resolve conflict, know who is in our ingroup, find a mate, reproduce, and raise children. Relationships bring us security, connection, joy, fun, love, and much more. They can also be a source of disconnection, loneliness, and much more. The quality of our relationships determines the quality of our lives.

Perspectives on Relationships

Here are a few perspective-taking skills that can help you in your relationships. A friend, relative, colleague, or partner has lots of different aspects, some that you like, some that make you laugh, others that you don't know about, and still others that you find annoying. In the same way that you befriend all the aspects of your own mind—the good, the bad, and the ugly—so too you can learn to step back and see others' layers, faults, and eccentricities. And maybe even what they felt, thought, and why they act the way they do. This is hard to do but is part of holding your own immediate judgments in check and seeing the bigger picture.

> SOPHIA: *When my mother's dementia had really taken hold, I learned that reasoning with her was not helpful. If I did, she'd get agitated or, even worse, paranoid. No amount of telling her she was safe in a residential home, that her husband had died a few years earlier, and that I was her oldest daughter reassured her. She couldn't really take in news of my life. I learned that when she was agitated what helped was brushing her hair, stroking her hand, giving her a foot rub—very physical things that she seemed to find soothing. In those moments I could see a part of her that was scared and wanted comforting; it was a part of her I'd not really seen before.*
>
> *Sometimes putting on some music she knew and singing together gave her a lot of joy. We'd sing together, and sometimes we'd get up and dance. I signed her up for the dance evenings in the residential home, which became a highlight of her week.*
>
> *At other times, when she was bright and in a good mood, we'd get out photo albums and reminisce about chapters in her life that she remembered vividly. In those moments she was happy. And I learned about parts of her life I had no idea about.*

When relationships become strained, it can be helpful to take a barometric check on our bodies and minds. Your chest, shoulders, neck, and face often provide a good readout of how you're doing. When you shut down or are fired up by feeling upset or angry, your perspective can become limited and limiting.

The first step here is to recognize what is happening and see what your body is trying to tell you.

So often we turn to problem solving in relationships. That may or may not be the right thing to do. Being able to observe what is happening not only in us but in a relationship opens the possibility of asking, "Is this a moment that requires thinking or experiencing or both?"

> SAM: *Nurse training, especially in places like ICUs and hospice care, often skimps on the human side of things. This memory of my first week in the ICU still haunts me. There was this man who called me over one evening, saying, "I am scared that if I fall asleep, I will never wake up. But I am in so much pain, I want to sleep." I wanted to help, and I thought he was asking for help with pain control. I rushed off to find my supervisor to discuss it, but when I got back less than 10 minutes later, he had died. I can't be certain, but my gut feeling is that he wanted me to hold his hand and talk to him while he drifted off. It hit me hard. From that point on, in moments like that I am going to listen to my gut and listen to what it is telling me.*

Being able to step back and move between experiencing, thinking, and observing can help us know "What is needed in this moment?" We'll return to this question in the next chapter.

Perspectives on Technology

People are often quick to blame cellphones, social media, and the Internet for all sorts of problems. It is doubtless true that many phone apps and games are designed to grab and keep our attention, driving it to places the developers want us to go and capturing as much information about us as they can. It may require a Herculean effort, but they can also be useful to us rather than the other way around. Anchoring yourself and trying to stay connected to your body can help you step back, keep you from getting sucked in, and use them only in ways you choose by staying connected to your values and intentions.

> SAM: *I can game like there is no tomorrow, and I have been known to pull all-nighters. But here's what I do now. I got this timer on my phone now, especially for work nights, got to cap my gaming. Don't get me wrong, I love gaming. It's how I connect with friends, get that buzz from competing, and some of the games are next-level real, it's unreal. But I need my sleep, especially workdays. So I got this app for when I am studying. Blocks out chunks of time and locks me out of everything else on my phone. It also throws some rewards for staying focused. It's like having my own coach.*

We're taking control of our technology; it is there to serve us.

Perspective and Culture

We are part of a wider ecosystem. The ground, air, weather, birds, animals, and other trees are part of any tree's ecosystem. In the same way, we are shaped by the wider culture in which we were raised and in which we live. This includes honoring and discrimination, inclusion and exclusion, equality and inequality in all their forms.

> SAM: *Growing up as a white boy in Botswana was incredible. It gave me this whole different perspective and helped me realize that there are different ways of living. Now coming out as gay, I'm super tuned in to where I feel like I belong and where I stand out from the crowd.*

> MOHAMMED: *I was born here, and I get asked all the time, "Where are you from?" When I say here, people get this look and sometimes ask, "No, where are you from originally?" As a young Muslim some people look at me with this look like "Is he safe?" I am used to it, but it's not okay. It can get into me, I question myself, I ask myself if I am okay.*

Discrimination and inequality create untold suffering and need to be addressed at every level. This includes in our practice and lives. Can you see moments where you feel excluded or different? Or where you create difference and exclusion? Can you respond with clarity and courage and use all that you've learned to respond wisely?

> MOHAMMED: *It is a work in progress, but my daughters are strong—they own who they are, have chosen good friends, and we talk a lot about what it is like for them to be brown and Muslim in a predominantly white and non-Muslim city. The other day a teacher asked one of them, "Where are you from?" and my daughter said, "That's a tricky question." I suspect the teacher felt a bit uncomfortable. We talked about it with my daughter when she got home and helped her work out an answer that works for her. She is Muslim and brown, her parents sought refuge and were granted asylum here, but she is so much more than that. I spoke to the teacher, and she asked if I would join the school parents' forum to help advise the school on its inclusion and equality policies.*

The Ancient Oak: On Authenticity

The writer, psychologist, and teacher Ram Dass suggested that we see ourselves and others as we see trees, more impersonally. There are different types, cherry, oak, pine. . . . Some are tiny, like bonsai, some huge, like conifers. Some are bent, and some of them stand tall, soaring upward. If a tree doesn't get enough light, it turns and grows toward the light. We don't get judgmental and reactive about it. We appreciate the tree.

Trees just are. We just are, similar and different, shaped by our circumstances. It can help to look at people this way, firmly rooted, growing toward the light, bent into their particular shape by all that's happened.

Perspective and Wise Action

When we act out of habit, reactively we're relying on all that we've learned to do the right thing. That's fine most of the time. But sometimes wise action requires stepping back to see the bigger picture. A powerful example is what happened in March 1968 when the village My Lai in Vietnam was subject to a horrific massacre. It was during the war between Vietnam and the United States, and a company of American soldiers killed hundreds of unarmed civilians, mostly women, older men, and children. The killing was ended by three Americans in command of a helicopter, led by 25-year-old Hugh Thompson, Jr. They were there to provide the infantry with cover against Viet Cong fighters. Thompson was only 25 years old, working alongside armed American infantry men, led by officers who outranked him, in a volatile and dangerous situation. As he flew over the scene, he couldn't see any Viet Cong fighters, even though there was a lot of shooting. When he realized there were no Viet Cong fighters and his fellow Americans were killing unarmed villagers, he landed his helicopter between the villagers and the soldiers. He trained his machine guns on the American soldiers and ordered his two crew members to open fire on the American infantry men if they further harmed the villagers. In those minutes Thompson's perspective of Us/Them, of hierarchy, and of how the army operated shifted. In the face of a frightening, fast-moving, and horrific scene he showed extraordinary courage. Those decisions saved many lives and curtailed further horrific massacre of villagers. But they cost him heavily in the years ahead, as many in the military took the perspective that his actions had betrayed his fellow soldiers and country.

Awareness

Normally what happens in moment-by-moment experience is that our foreground and awareness are either absent or in the background. Identifying with thoughts and images means being lost in them, we have this sense of being carried away by our thoughts, or maybe we have a sliver of awareness—"I'm thinking" or "These are my thoughts." But this moment of identification is a trick of perception.

Perspective is about reversing this. Bringing awareness into the foreground allows you to see your moment-by-moment experiences from a wider viewpoint. The stories you tell yourself about what you're doing, what's happening, the "blah, blah, blah," quiets down. Standing back and observing from a different point of view is the beginning of awareness.

In full-blown awareness, there is lucid, luminescent seeing and understanding. Even observing can become part of moment-by-moment experiencing. When this happens, we can even lose a sense of identifying with what's happening. Instead of "I am meditating, that's my heartbeat, this is interesting, oh no, my mind just wandered," there is simply a sense of experience unfolding moment by moment: "hearing bird song, thinking, sensing heartbeat, feeling warmth." This can involve a sense of connection, stillness, and expansiveness; "I," time, and space can even fall away. At first this kind of awareness is quite fleeting. But this fleeting awareness hints that this is available to us. With practice it's something you can start to access more. It can teach us a lot, because we can experience how our mind and body create and re-create experience moment to moment, but with a real sense of being close to and observing the experience. If this all sounds like a lot, that's okay; it is a lifelong practice.

Perhaps this sounds a bit mystical, but it's not meant to be. You are cultivating the conditions for your mindfulness practice to be a teacher, so you can experience for yourself how your mind creates and re-creates experience and start to play an active role toward a mind—and life—that is in line with your values and aspirations. You don't have to be the person you believe you should be. Your sense of self is a process, impossible to pin down with any one definition. The same can be true of how you see others and the world around you. The minute you label others, you make it harder to see other aspects of who they can be.

The Ancient Oak: It's Not Meant to Be Mystical

Saying "It's not meant to be mystical" does not devalue the experience of people who are drawn to the spiritual, mystical, or sacred aspects of contemplative practices. What is being offered is a way of being, of opening to a different way of knowing, in which what you choose to explore is up to you. For example, many people use mindfulness practices in their religious traditions, as a way of being fully present and open. What these practices offer is a way of being aware, open, and responsive, not only in our everyday life but also potentially in other, more spiritual, or religious areas of our lives, such as in prayer, contemplation, or service.

TROUBLESHOOTING: Changing Perspective

Stepping back and *changing perspective is sometimes misunderstood as being detached, disconnected, or standoffish.* It is far from that—we remain close to, intimate with our moment-by-moment unfolding experience, but we're observing and befriending it.

Tripping into rumination or fantasy. At any stage of this work of learning to shift perspective, we can resort to habit or trip into reactivity. We can get hopeless or worried when shifting into the past or future, inviting the perspective of someone else can lead to feeling more or less than, and so on. Rumination, worry, catastrophizing, self-justification, doom scrolling, and many habits can all, at their worst, be very powerful, like being dragged into a vortex. The laws of physics speak of an equal or greater force needed to pull us out of this force. In some senses that is right. Sometimes grounding requires a storm anchor, using something that is up to the task. But sometimes a small shift can change the whole dynamic. A kayaker being dragged toward Niagara Falls can with some light, skillful paddle strokes find a back eddy or use the current to get to the riverbank. The key is to see all of this as part of the practice, bringing interest to what's happened, and then, like the kayaker, steadying and anchoring yourself.

Taking a Different Viewpoint for Life

Astronauts have often related what it's like to look down at earth from space. They describe witnessing the planet from that distance with its 7 billion people and how small yet beautiful it is in the vastness of space. They have described it as a powerful thought, but also as a direct, emotional experience—an experiential knowing, a sense of this earth being our home. We don't all have to go to space to be able to do this. As Oscar Wilde put it, "We are all in the gutter, but some of us are looking at the stars."

The ability to take a different viewpoint creates the space to stop and ask, "What is happening?" From this viewpoint it is more possible to recognize and allow difficult experiences that may previously have tipped into automatic, understandable reactions or just felt overwhelming. It is also possible to recognize and savor good experiences that previously we may have glossed over. It creates a space in which it's possible to choose how to respond in any given moment, a theme we turn to in the next chapter.

9

Responding Wisely

Between stimulus and reaction, there is a space.
In that space is moment-by-moment awareness
In that moment we can choose our response.

What would be your immediate reaction to the scenarios below?

A momentary sadness . . .

A notification on your phone of a message from a good friend . . .

Someone speaking to you in a disrespectful way . . .

These are everyday moments in the countless stream of moments that make up every day. Mostly we barely register them, and even if we do, our reaction is automatic. So far, you have learned to:

- Gather, stabilize. and anchor your attention
- Recognize and start to better understand what's happening in your mind and body
- Befriend your mind and meet whatever comes up with interest, kindness, and care
- Take different perspectives

Steady attention shines light on the unfolding processes of our minds. Awareness with an attitude of friendliness makes everything seem more possible. This groundwork creates the possibility that, instead of reacting automatically, you can choose how you respond. Instead of asking "Why do I feel this way?" you ask yourself, "What does this moment need?" Seeing what is happening in our minds and bodies, stepping back from reactivity, and choosing our responses is the focus of this chapter.

Learning to Respond Wisely in Life

MOHAMMED: *My wife and I took a weekend away recently, just the two of us. It was the first holiday my wife had had for a while, and she really needed it. We had to take a three-hour ferry ride to the island where we were going, and when we got aboard my wife said, "Look, there is Wi-Fi. I am going to just finish up my work." She saw a shadow cross my face, and we held our gaze for a second. She's always compulsively working, and I tend not to say what I want and then go quiet—sulk, I guess. In that moment as we held each other's eye, we both knew that's what we do, and we had a chance to do something different. She, to her credit, said, "Mohammed, sorry, we really need this time together. Let's go on deck and enjoy the sun and view. You sleep late tomorrow morning, and I will finish up my work then."*

Responding wisely involves first recognizing what is happening, then creating a pause, and then in that pause you have a chance to do something different: respond wisely. The more you do this, the more you grow your capacity to respond wisely.

PRACTICE: **Responding Wisely**

You can follow along on our website.

This practice develops the capacity for responding wisely. You start by steadying and grounding yourself, softening and relaxing any areas of tension and your mind, and anchoring in your body. Then you bring to mind something that is causing you some difficulty but feels manageable. Then, intentionally, take a Three-Step Breathing Space, and from this place of being anchored and with an attitude of friendly interest and care, see what comes up in response to these questions:

- "What would be a helpful response?"
- "What would support my well-being?"
- "What would support the well-being of others?"

What comes up? See if you can trust what emerges in your body, and if nothing comes up, see if you can hold a sense of not knowing, with patience.

What can you learn in this practice? First, that you can notice body sensations, emotions, impulses, and thoughts in real time, even when something difficult is happening. Second, that the Three-Step Breathing Space helps you first note, then anchor and shift to an experiential way of knowing. This can open creative, flexible, and resilient responses.

LING: *I have done a lot of work on what triggers me. Don't get me wrong, I love my kids. But I struggle when they are moody or, worse still, rude. I can easily snap, and then things get out of hand. This pause makes all the difference—in it I see my rising irritation and impulse to snap. What was helpful? Self-talk like "Ling, you're the grown-up here." Holding back and then choosing my moment. Putting myself in their shoes; I was their age once. And being kind to myself. I am a single parent of teenagers; that's hard for everyone.*

This approach can be applied equally to any situation where you think it can be helpful to pause and ask, "What would be helpful here?" This can be moments of happiness, anxiety, humor, indecision, beauty, guilt, love, or loneliness. It can be people or situations that trigger us. It may be wider issues in the world that preoccupy us, like climate change. At these moments, you can make it a habit to pause, note what is happening, anchor in your bodies, and then consider, "What does this moment need? What would be a helpful response?"

The Breathing Space is an everyday, mini version of the responding wisely practice. It helps you pause, anchor, and shift perspective. It is the same Breathing Space that you learned in Chapter 3, but here you are using it intentionally in moments of reactivity and at the end you are asking yourself:

- "What does this moment need?"
- "What would be a helpful response?"
- "What would support my well-being?"
- "What would support the well-being of others in this situation?"

LING: *When I started to integrate this practice into my life, I realized how much of each day I am in survival mode. My work as a court reporter, single-parenting my kids, dealing with their dad, my ex, taking care of the house, the car, the cat. There are so many moments that stress me out and that I normally just survive. But more and more, on a good day, I'm learning I don't need to keep paddling like crazy; sometimes I can stow the paddles and go with the flow.*

Where the Responding Wisely practice helps you develop the capacity for being less reactive, the mini version offers you *the possibility of responding wisely in challenging moments.*

The Ancient Oak: Possibilities

The philosopher Søren Kierkegaard wrote about this moment of choice.

"If I were to wish for anything, I should not wish for wealth and power, but for the passionate sense of the potential, for the eye which, ever young and ardent, sees the possible. Pleasure disappoints, possibility never. And what wine is so sparkling, what so fragrant, what so intoxicating, as possibility!"

The space that present moment awareness creates is this moment of possibility, a pause that enables us to see the different doorways through which we can go.

Different Doorways to Responding Wisely: Noticing Reactivity

When you pause, you have an opportunity to notice that you are in a moment of reactivity. You can open new possibilities of responding by choosing a doorway to walk through to discover what is happening in this moment. What you discover may lead you to respond in a different way, more wisely, but it is just the first step.

The Body Door

You've seen how the body can be an anchor and a different way of being. In Step 3 of the Breathing Space you floodlight your body with awareness. The body is one possible doorway you can walk through, where you can choose to stay with awareness of your body, riding the waves of whatever is happening there. You start to know what the body needs—perhaps some deep breaths, some stretches, a walk, a drink or some food, a physical connection, a hug, sexuality.

> LING: *When I am wired and tired after a long day, my body is wound up tightly like a coil. I may even have neck and back pain or even a headache. What do I need in these moments? I've learned breathing, shoulder rolls, shaking out my arms and legs, and changing my posture to something more like my favorite massive yew tree than a gnarly shrub (smiling). I try to stay tuned in as I deliberately work on loosening body tension with my breath and movements and coming home to my strong and ever-present body. It is empowering.*

Many people start to describe their body as somewhere to always come home to, a safe place, even a sanctuary.

The Mindfulness Practice Door

In any moment of awareness, one option is to drop into mindfulness practice. The active choice you are making is to take some time for yourself and see what you become aware of that you had not seen (smelled, tasted, felt, heard, etc.) while you were rushing to react. As your mindfulness practice develops, you will have more of a sense of what practice you need in that moment. This could be some breathing, walking, movement practice, or a Breathing Space.

> LING: *If I wake up in the night and start worrying, I do a Body Scan. Nine times out of ten I am asleep before I get to my torso.*

The Thoughts Doorway

Through this doorway you're observing your thoughts, but from a different perspective. You're able to see them as thoughts and not facts. It can help to label thoughts, especially if it's an old familiar pattern. Sometimes the thoughts or images merge into a whole pattern. It can help to give the thoughts a name or write them down, so you can see them on paper. Naming and writing down thoughts creates a pause and helps with perspective. Take care to ensure you're talking to yourself as a good friend helps. "I'm jumping to conclusions; slow down." "That's my inner critic talking; pipe down." "I've got this."

The Wise Action Doorway

The question "What will support me and others?" is intended to bypass over-thinking and allow answers to come up more intuitively. It could be an act of self-care, doing something pleasurable, something that gives you a sense of achievement, or an action that addresses the situation.

The Reentry Doorway

The Breathing Space also offers a doorway that I'll call *reentry*. Here you go back to whatever you were doing before but having "reset." You may be stepping back into the same situation, *but you've changed.*

These doorways are just a few that people find helpful as they start this work of intentionally noticing moments of reactivity and developing the possibility of responding wisely.

Broadening and Building Wise Responding

Befriending your mind by cultivating the attitudes of mindfulness (Chapter 7) reveals, opens, and even widens doorways. Curiosity infuses any moment with a spirit of "Isn't this interesting?" and "I wonder what will happen." Through appreciation you learn what you value and enjoy, so that these doorways open to you. Openness and courage ensure you are open to possibilities that you might not ordinarily consider and help you be brave enough to try walking through them. Letting go helps you avoid the dead ends you might have walked into out of habit. When you have a sense of your mind as your friend, wise responding becomes so much easier.

SOPHIA: *I was in my living room this week with my grandson, Noah, and Rufus, my dog. Noah was playing with his trucks, and Rufus was asleep in his bed. I had put the mug on the arm of the chair where I was sitting because my tremors were quite bad, but it crashed to the floor. The tea spilled and the mug's handle broke. Rufus looked up from his bed, came over to see what had happened, sniffed the liquid to see if it was worth drinking, decided no, and then went back to his bed. Noah looked on with delight at the whole scene—the noise, the cup breaking, the spill, my reaction, and Rufus's reaction. He came over as well to explore the situation in much the same way, although he used his hands to explore the liquid, mug, and broken handle. It was interesting: neither Rufus nor Noah reacted the way I instinctively had, berating myself—"You stupid idiot."*

I am not sure I'll ever fully shake off my inner critic. As the mug fell and smashed into pieces, it was as though time slowed down and I felt the shame and horror wash through me like a tsunami. Not just my mind, but my body too.

But this time I got interested in how Rufus and Noah reacted. Noah's parents, my daughter and son-in-law, are balanced and caring; Noah hasn't internalized the same self-critic I have. He was just curious, even joyful about this interesting experience. All three of us in this little scene—Noah, Rufus, and I—had an initial experience as our attention was drawn to the spill and broken mug. As I've learned, that was the first arrow. My mind was ready to fire a volley of second arrows stemming from the wave of shame and I had learned growing up: "I should behave perfectly. Making mistakes means I am stupid."

Even though an arrow or two were fired, I chose to get down on the ground with Noah. It was a wood floor, so no harm had been done. I want Noah to have good memories of me. And, more than that, I want him to be happy, without being crippled by the inner critic that has been part of me for so long. Moments like this suggest he will have this gift, which gives me great joy. I mostly did okay with my son, but Noah seems so together, so happy—that gives me great joy.

Knowing How Our Frame of Mind Shapes How We Respond

Our frame of mind primes our reactions and choices. It is important to recognize the emotional states (tiredness, sadness, anxiety, shame, anger) most likely to prime reactivity and poor choices.

> ### The Barefoot Professor: How Our State of Mind Shapes Reactivity
>
> In his book *Thinking Fast and Slow*, the Nobel Prize-winning psychologist Daniel Kahneman explains how we respond to situations is in part determined by shortcuts called "heuristics." Heuristics are rules of thumb that help us make sense of the world, simplify complex information, and make quick decisions. They can take many forms but might involve approximating to prototypical situations (representativeness heuristic) and looking for information to verify what we already believe (confirmation heuristic). Heuristics help us manage information overload; we simply can't process everything that is happening. But many studies now show that negative emotions like fear and anger trigger particular heuristics. Perhaps this was functional in our distant evolutionary story. At times of threat we don't have the luxury of thinking things through; a quick reaction might be the difference between surviving and not surviving. In a social situation, where the dynamics mean we might be about to be excluded from the group, de-escalating conflict or seeking shelter is needed.
>
> On the other hand, positive emotions, like joy and contentment, expand our sense of what is possible. We're less likely to jump to some of our shortcuts. The implications are important. Can we better understand and see these shortcuts (heuristics) and know when they serve and when they don't? Can we cultivate these more positive emotions, not only because they're pleasurable, but because they resource us? They make it more possible to deal with challenges and to live our lives more fully?

While our state of body and mind prime our reactions, there are some ways to start moving away from reactivity. The first, which we've already covered, is to become more aware of moments of reactivity and in doing so to see the different doorways available in these moments. The second is to realize which states of body and mind make us more likely to be reactive—typically negative states like anger and, riding out these moments, taking care of us, avoiding situations that might trigger reactivity. This is much of what the next few chapters will help you with.

Third, I have emphasized cultivating certain attitudes of mind and positive emotions because they make reactivity less likely and resource us to respond wisely. This could be the difference between saying and doing things we later regret versus holding our tongue, putting off important choices for when we're in a better position to make them, and acting in ways that align with our values.

Learning anything new requires practice, and to get good at it you need to practice in more and more pressured settings. Here are some questions that may help you in moments of potential reactivity.

- How could I respond to myself like a good friend?
- In the past, what has helped in moments of reactivity?
- What has enabled me to move from reacting to responding?
- What about when the going gets tough—what's helped me then?
- How could I best care for myself at these times?
- How could I respond to the turmoil of thoughts and feelings without adding to them?
- Where is a safe place, both literally but also in my mind?

LING: *I often have a word with myself; self-talk is good. It's hard for me, but I try to accept help, trust others, and trust myself.*

SOPHIA: *A hug, from my grandson or partner. I let go of perfection. I am learning I quite like to take a nap. I love going for walks with my dog, Rufus.*

MOHAMMED: *Self-control and choosing to be courageous, even if I feel scared. I learned that through sports.*

SAM: *My ninja of course.*

What are your answers? Maybe you could form an intention to use these the next time you face this challenging situation and see what happens.

TROUBLESHOOTING: Responding Wisely to Common Obstacles

Change isn't easy. But we know quite a lot about what supports change. Here are some tips.

Start with small steps. As with any new skill, you're most likely to learn and develop confidence if you start with something small and manageable. The expression "couch to 5K" refers to all the steps required to build the fitness to run a 5K. You're more likely to progress and use other questions. The questions are intended to open a sense of possibility.

Take the long view. This work takes time and is supported by your mindfulness practice and the ways in which you integrate it into your life. Don't expect overnight change.

Revise or replace the questions. If the questions "What does this moment need?" and "What will support my well-being?" don't seem quite right in a given situation, trust yourself and use other questions. The questions are intended to open a sense of possibility.

> SOPHIA: *Every time I have moved, I have packed up my house and decided what to take to my new home. After the divorce I downsized, and so had to let a lot of stuff go, everything we had accumulated as a family. I became paralyzed with indecision. I used a question Marie Kondo, the Japanese writer, suggests for decluttering: asking with each item, "Does this spark joy?" That question after a Breathing Space was perfect; it made it so clear what I wanted to keep. Then with the pile of things to let go, I asked again, "Can any of these things spark joy for others?" There were children's toys, clothing, some furniture. Here the answer was often "yes." That was great, as I found ways to recycle a lot of the stuff. I loved the idea of the three piles: keep, which bring me joy; recycle, which might bring others joy; and let go.*

Responding Wisely in Real Life, for Life

Throughout our lives it is inevitable that we will live through upsetting and distressing times. To cope with stress and go about our day effectively, responding wisely to difficult moments, it is helpful to have a sense of what we can manage and what might overwhelm us—our window of tolerance. Your window of tolerance is the level of bodily arousal at which you can know what you're feeling, can think clearly, and are able to solve problems. But if we are overstimulated, these abilities are lost, and we become overwhelmed. This can manifest as heart racing; sweatiness; intrusive images; confusion; feeling on edge, scared, or panicky; extreme emotions; or mood swings. Conversely, we can shut down. This can manifest as tuning out, experiencing numbness, being unable to think, feeling cut off from others, dissociated, flat, or low.

> The key is to know the window in which it is possible for you to respond wisely. And if you're outside that window, what you need to do to take care of yourself.

Responding wisely is really only possible in your window of tolerance. Outside it, we just don't function well or at all.

The Barefoot Professor:
Trauma and Posttraumatic Stress

The times when our sense of safety, sense of self, and ability to cope is severely challenged or even overwhelmed are called *traumatic stress*. It can have lasting effects, which is called *posttraumatic stress*. Almost anything can be traumatic, from emotional abuse to domestic violence to the many forms of sexual abuse to medical procedures to accidents and natural disasters. Some people experience long-term trauma over months or even years, such as those seeking asylum from war-torn countries or those raised in a family where violence was a daily occurrence. It can be low level and chronic, working in a work environment marked by high levels of criticism, harassment, and pressure, with little or no support. Others can experience a one-off trauma, like a car accident. Typically, trauma undermines our capacity to feel safe, our sense of being able to cope and to form loving relationships. This is because at a bodily level it heightens our sensitivity to threat and affects our ability to self-soothe. In extreme forms we can experience posttraumatic stress disorder, where the traumatic memories live on as intrusive thoughts and nightmares, constantly being reexperienced, as if they were happening again and again. This is very upsetting, so people start to become very avoidant, not only of what triggers these memories but sometimes of emotions altogether.

A history of trauma and posttraumatic stress disorder severely limits our window of tolerance because intrusive memories and scary bodily sensations can easily be activated and sometimes stay in place for days, weeks, or even longer.

If a mindfulness practice tends to trigger you out of your window of tolerance and you know or worry that you have posttraumatic stress disorder, listen to what your experience is telling you and seek professional help. Trust yourself; don't do anything that your experience tells you is not helpful.

Everyone is different, shaped by our genetics, childhood, life experiences, and current life situation. But crucially, mindfulness practices such as gathering and anchoring our awareness, grounding, and befriending can all broaden our window of tolerance. You can build your capacity in small ways by practicing with your eyes open, working with your breath intentionally to regulate your arousal, taking a few deeper inbreaths and slower outbreaths, doing only what you know you can manage, and self-soothing in ways you know work for you. More than this, the context of any moment, how well you slept, how safe you feel in any moment, also affect the window of tolerance.

LING: *I have learned when I am triggered to feel my feet touching the ground and the places in my body that are calm. I can recognize the column of tightness and contraction in my torso that is fear and the tears of anger that well up in these moments. I am learning that these are moments in which I can steady myself enough to do what I need to take care of myself. Sometimes I wrestle my demons, sometimes I dance with them, and sometimes I snuggle with them. And I finally worked up the courage to make some changes in my life.*

Being the Change We Want to See in the World

I can't breathe. Please, please, please. I can't breathe.

These were the last words of George Floyd, an African American murdered in May 2020 by a white policeman in Minneapolis. The policeman, Derek Chauvin, was "restraining" him by holding his boot on his neck and asphyxiating him. There was global condemnation, and riots erupted in cities across America, but also throughout the world.

MOHAMMED: *As I watched the news, tears of anger and helplessness ran down my face. I not only felt for him, but I could identify with the discrimination, injustice, fear, and hatred that were playing out on the news. As I sat there in front of my TV, I tried to steady myself by connecting with my roots—strong, steady, able to flex with the storm that was playing out around the world.*

What happened as I did that? A sense that my anger about the hatred and police brutality—no, murder—could be channeled into something positive. I had to speak and act in ways that create the very world I want to see for myself, but more importantly for my children. That evening, instead of reading to my kids, I found a way to tell them about George Floyd. I also told them about some of my experiences and where my parents fled from in fear of their lives, wanting somewhere safe for their children. We talked about their dreams, and that their dreams mattered; their strengths and potential, which deserve to be seen and allowed to develop; and that they should walk through their days tall, without having to worry about what others might say or do because of their religion or the color of their skin or the fact that they were girls. My daughter said that she was angry because the boys sometimes didn't let her play soccer with them. I said, "Yes, I understand you feel frustrated and angry, and I want you to feel hopeful, because we're going to make things better, we're going change this. Everyone deserves the same chances in life." This was the first of many conversations that were woven into our family and the way my wife and I chose to raise our children.

We can expand on how we started the chapter:

Between stimulus and reaction, there is a space
In that space is moment-by-moment awareness
In that moment we can choose how we respond
With our response we shape our lives and the world.

The Ancient Oak and the Barefoot Professor: How the Wider World Shapes Our Experience

The Ancient Oak: Our response is framed by the realities of our wider lives; choices that are and are not available to us because of our social and economic status, our sex, our gender identity, our cultural background, the color of our skin, our age, and so on. It is naïve to neglect how important this is. In fact, it is probably the place to start with any wise action. When trying to understand why someone behaves the way they do, rather than saying "That's who they are," pause and ask, "What is this person coming to this moment with, in terms of their place in life and all that they have learned? What possibilities are available to them?" If a child comes to school lethargic, perhaps it is because they share a bedroom in a small house and they have had no breakfast.

The Barefoot Professor: Psychology research has shown that we tend to attribute our successes to ourselves and our failures to our circumstances. But we reverse that for other people; they get lucky when good things happen, but they're responsible when things go wrong. Of course, it is likely that most of the time it is a combination of the two, framed by the wider context.

Every day you are faced with choices about what you say and do. The anger at George Floyd's murder rippled through the world. The example of Mohammed and his daughters is how such events can play out for ordinary people. The way he responded and talked to his daughters is how hope and change are enacted. History teaches us that collective and persistent action can create change. But it would be naïve to think that change in wider systems is easy.

Throughout your days and life you have the chance to respond wisely to the myriad moments you navigate at home, at work, in relationships, and the wider world. These moments may be small, such as how you respond to the smile of an elderly neighbor, or large, like the decisions you make at key transition points in your life. Your opportunities to respond wisely extend also to the issues in the wider world that affect you and that you can in your own way change, such as hatred, discrimination, inequality, injustice, and climate change. And of course, these wider issues will require collective commitment and effort by human minds and hearts.

Every moment is important because these moments make up your day. The accumulation of all these moments makes up your life. If you respond wisely in these moments, you shape the course of your life. If you shape the course of your life, you shape the world.

The Ancient Oak: Taking Action

More than 2,000 years ago Epictetus was born into slavery but became one of the great Greek philosophers. His essential idea was we may not be able to control our circumstances, but we remain responsible for our actions. Here is an example of his teaching.

> Caretake this moment.
> Immerse yourself in its particulars.
> Respond to this person, this challenge, this deed.
> Quit evasions.
> Stop giving yourself needless trouble.
> It is time to really live; to fully inhabit the situation you happen to be in now.

A more recent example is Edith Eger, who was incarcerated as a child in a concentration camp. She wrote, "But even then, in my prison, I could choose how I responded, I could choose my actions and speech, I could choose what I held in my mind."

And finally, a contemporary example is Greta Thunberg, who has made climate change her life's mission.

Our Values Are Our Compass

We ask children, "What do you want to be when you grow up?" How can they know? We say, "Follow your dream." But often people think, "I don't know what that means" or "That's unrealistic. I have commitments, financially, to other people." Pausing and asking questions about our lives can also easily create the very judgments that cause misery: "if only . . . ," "I should . . . ," "I ought . . . ," and so on.

Navigation involves having a sense of where we're trying to get to and using a compass to stay on track. Inevitably we go off track, but the compass helps us keep going in the right direction. Our values act as that compass; they are our true north.

What Is Important to Me? What Do I Value? What Is My True North?

You can follow along on our website.

This exercise is designed to help you identify your values. Normally, values are deeply held beliefs that guide your actions, the sort of person you want to be, how you'd like to be in relation to other people and the world. Everyone's values are different—your values are your values, and they can evolve over time. It can help to create an event in your mind, one where people would come and celebrate you in some way. This could be a big birthday party (your 16th, 18th, 21st, 30th, any year you choose) or a gathering that marks some transition, like starting or leaving a job, a retirement party. What you do is choose people whose opinion you care about (your partner, good friends, family, mentors, a teacher, colleagues) and ask yourself if they were to speak about you at this event what might they say they like and respect about you.

     You might like to store whatever you come up with on your phone or write them down. These values are the compass that gives you direction, including when you are off track. You use your values, in the space between stimulus and response, to know what a wise response is. They turn a blueprint into something real.

SOPHIA: *At my 70th birthday, I'd like my children to say, "She was there for me when I needed her." This helps me. If I have a choice, I always put them first. My partner says I am a pushover, but he values his freedom and I value my kids, even though they have grown and flown the nest.*

If you want to take this exercise further, you could consider what these people might say about how you were in your work, your community, and the wider world. These values are about the impact we have on the people around us and our wider world.

SAM: *When I qualify as a specialist ICU nurse, I'd like my patients to say, "He always kept his human touch." I'd like my friends to say, "He was a good laugh."*

How do values translate into wise action? By action I mean what we say, what we do, and just as important, what we don't say and don't do.

In response to George Floyd's murder, Mohammed decided to channel his energy in several ways, through the people in his immediate circle, especially his daughters and how he raised them. He joined several of the protest marches in his city and connected with some groups similarly interested in addressing racism and injustice in his local community as part of the Black Lives Matter movement. He decided that every time he experienced hatred or discrimination in his life going forward this would be a chance to pause and ask, "What does this moment need? What would be helpful to me, to others, and to the wider world?"

Our values pervade our being and all that we do, whether we're aware of it or not. As we are social, this includes the values of those around us and the collective values of our family, workplace, or community. Being part of these groups means being aware and sensitive to others' values, both those we share and those that are different.

> **The Barefoot Professor: Shared Values**
>
> Social identity researchers have shown that a large part of how we see ourselves has to do with whatever larger social groups we are part of. This can be a religion, occupation, nationality, sexual orientation, ethnic group, or gender identity. It shapes many aspects of life, who we regard as "us" and who as "them," work opportunities, access to education, and so on. Social identity includes identifying with our group's values, so our true north is as much our group's true north.

Our values are important because they guide us to our true north. That means that bringing awareness to our minds, bodies, and actions reveals when we are on course and when we've deviated. If at the end of the day you put your head on the pillow and you have a sense of peace, more than likely your day was one in which your actions and values lined up. This can be true even if the day was full of frustrations and difficulties; if you feel you kept your true north in those moments, then a sense of ease can prevail. On the other hand, agitation, disquiet, guilt, and anger may be pointing to our lives and values being out of sync.

Taking the Responding Wisely Practice Further

Responding wisely can be practiced for a lifetime. First, you can respond to the full range of experience, be it pleasant or unpleasant, good or bad, pleasurable or aversive, significant or trivial, boring or exciting. In all these moments, try asking, with curiosity, kindness, and care:

What is this?

If I really stop to tune in to my body, what is it telling me?

If I zoom out and take a different perspective, what do I see?

SAM: *When I'm at a club, or gig or bar, I am just out, having fun. But sometimes out of the blue, I get this random thought: "hell yes, life is fun."*

SOPHIA: *The moment when the cup of hot tea shattered on the floor and spilled every-where, there was so much going on in that moment, for me, for Noah, even for Rufus [smiling].*

LING: *When I lose my rag with my kids, I know deep down what it is about. When I was their age, I was in foster care. If I acted out, the way they do sometimes, I would get moved to new foster parents. I didn't have someone to rail against. I feel like shouting at my kids, "You don't know how lucky you are." But of course, they don't; they have had a different upbringing from mine. I'm proud of myself for that.*

The space before you respond provides an extraordinary opportunity. A good friend knows when to accept us, when to let us be, when to jolly us along, and when we need honest feedback. An attitude of curiosity, appreciation, kindness, courage, and care can broaden and deepen these spaces. Can you come up close to what you discover in these moments and be real and honest with yourself before responding? The more you can do this, the more your responses will be authentic.

LING: *The appreciation practice has shown me I have many good moments throughout the day. But my wrecking ball often comes in to destroy them with "I don't deserve this," "This won't last," "This isn't real," and so on and on. Naming, seeing, and stepping back enables me to see the thoughts and say, "Ha, wrecking ball, there you go, I'll just let you swing past, whoosh."*

SOPHIA: *When I was a teacher, I was good at my job, and the children, colleagues, and parents knew it. I worked hard to make sure my days were made up of good classes, where kids had fun and learned, my interactions with students were positive, and my conversations with parents constructive. But I rarely paused in these moments. I suppose I thought this is just what I do, and to do less would be to fail at my job. If I got compliments, I'd brush them off. I think people started to avoid complimenting me because I'd react like they were out of line. When I really examined these moments up close, I saw first my inner critic. But when I looked closely, I saw the inner critic was a house of cards. When it collapses, what is left is someone who really cares about her work, about the kids, their learning, their lives. Who loves that they appreciate what I do.*

MOHAMMED: *When the kids were tiny, I'd go into their room before I went to bed and make sure they were okay. One night I stood there for a while. I looked at one of the children, and in that moment, I had the thought "I don't actually like you." I was quite shocked; that's not a nice thought, and not one I expected. I sat down and did a Breathing Space, and the body door was the door that opened. What I found was bone-tiredness and fear, gripping my chest. I searched for a word, and it was resentment—that my days were so unrelenting with child care and fear that I wasn't up to it, that I wouldn't be able to be a good dad to this girl, who is different from me, she doesn't like sports and is arty and into books.*

SAM: *After breaking up with my partner, one of the first things I did was jump back into the dating app scene. To be real, it is more of a hookup app. I hooked up with a guy the same day I broke up with my partner. "To hell with my ex," I figured, "I'm single again." I enjoyed the thrill, the sex, being desired. But it left me feeling lonely. Most of the guys just want sex—duh, I guess that's what the app is for. I'd used the sex to try to feel less rejected and lonely.*

Often the questions "What does this moment need?" and "What would be a helpful response?" are enough. But you might like to try some other questions at these moments:

- What would enlarge me?
- What would enlarge others?
- What does my wisest/most compassionate/most courageous/friendliest voice have to say just now?
- If I were my own best friend/mentor/own parent, what would I suggest?
- What is the best outcome I can imagine?
- What feels true and authentic?

What comes up? Now ask:

How does this sit with me? Will I feel good about acting or not acting this way tomorrow, next year, at the end of my life? Will I regret acting or not acting this way?

What assumptions am I making? What am I expecting to happen? If I let go of these assumptions and expectations, what happens?

Of course, this is easier said than done. But in a way it is exactly like mindfulness of the breath. Minds wander. Being able to notice this and with firm kindness escorting the mind back is part of mindfulness practice. In the same way, sometimes you're carried away by reactivity, being able to notice this and with kindness, care, and patience coming back to this moment to start again. This work is lifelong and can support you in leading the life you aspire to.

SAM: *After my last relationship, I bellyflopped into a very deep hole. For weeks, I was dealing with dizziness, nausea, lightheadedness, feeling drained, and this overwhelming sensation that my world was closing in on me. What we had was real. How could it all just end? The thought crept in: "Will I ever find love again?"*

This wasn't my first time with these feelings. I had fallen into a similar hole when I was a teenager, around 15 or 16. Back then it was really confusing and felt so unknown. I had no idea if I'd get out and even less how to get out. Took a few months, but somehow I clambered out of that hole.

Then it happened again in my early 20s, and this time I had a sense of "Uh-oh, not this again." But this time the fear wasn't as paralyzing. I'd been here before, and by now I knew it had to do with my sexuality and feeling lonely and disconnected.

It took some time and lots of long talks with a good friend who gives great relationship advice. She shared a poem with me written by Portia Nelson, "Autobiography in Five Chapters." The poem is about someone falling into a hole repeatedly, like me, and figuring out first how to clamber out of the hole and then how to walk around the holes. I kind of knew what I needed to do. To get out of this hole I needed to come out to my parents and friends as gay.

But here I am again, in my mid-20s now. I know how I ended up here, and it's familiar, and I know it will pass. The last chapter of Portia Nelson's poem talks about walking down a different street. I have done my fair share of hookups now. I am ready for a relationship, with someone who sees me.

Being in a hole, as described in Portia Nelson's poem, is doubtless a dark and bleak place. But it can be understood as a time of withdrawal out of which can come a new perspective on our lives. Perhaps a problematic relationship or a draining work situation drives us into a hole. Perhaps our own habits, including habits of mind, are locking us in. Responding wisely at these times can be the difference between languishing and well-being.

> **PRACTICE:** **Falling in Holes, Walking around Holes, or Walking Down a Different Street?**
>
> Using Portia Nelson's poem to help us respond wisely.
>
> - In any moment, where are you now, walking down a well-maintained and lit street with a sense of confidence, walking down a street avoiding numerous potholes, traveling faster than is safe or in a hole?
> - What holes do you tend to fall down? How come?
> - What do you need to avoid falling into those holes?
> - What would walking down a different street look like for you?
> - What would it be like to walk down that street? What would you be doing and saying?
> - What skills and qualities do you need to walk that street? Courage, patience, interest, and trust? Does that feel possible? What would make it possible?

Portia Nelson's poem points to a sense of understanding colored with compassion that helps us begin to see these experiences afresh, walk around the holes, and in time perhaps even walk down different streets.

Wise Speech

For us human beings, words are one of our most powerful actions. With words we can connect, console, be consoled, create laughter, teach, learn, share news, and confide our hopes and fears. We can also criticize, divide, hurt, humiliate, lie, and withhold. Our speech, what we say and choose not to say, can be a powerful form of wise action.

Many contemplative and religious traditions offer guidance about speech. Typically, they suggest that we try to speak the truth, be kind, say only what is helpful, and consider the timing and impact of our words on others. Often they also include guidance on what not to say, which is in many cases the reverse of the qualities above, but includes speaking in ways that are grandiose, put others down, are coercive, dishonest, or vacuous.

By anchoring us in our bodies and listening to what our bodies have to say the 50–50 practice supports wise speech (Chapter 3, pages 64–67; Chapter 10, pages 199–200). Intentionally creating pauses when you're in company enables you to stay aware of what is being said with both words and body language. This is especially important if you're talking about something important or sensitive or when it is important that you make yourself understood. This requires clear language and courage.

When you speak, there can be moments where you don't know what to say. Being able to recognize and allow these moments can be a very powerful communication. You're giving one another space, to listen to your body and see ideas shifting. We were a social species long before we had language; we're always communicating even when we're not talking. If you notice an impulse to fill the space with words, see if you can practice nonreactivity. Perhaps you can check in with what is important to you, your values, and under your breath asking the questions about the right thing to say in this moment. Out of this might come something you hadn't anticipated.

> SAM: As a nurse I do this all the time because it is important to me. There are times when how I am with a patient or family member speaks louder than any words I could say. Being present and coming across as calm can be incredibly reassuring, especially when people are scared and overwhelmed. I try to nurse in a way that helps patients feel safe and reassured, whether it's checking vitals, inserting drips, changing dressings—whatever I'm doing. Patients die on the ICU, and when the doctor has told them this is likely to happen, we need to stay steady for those patients and their families. Some patients don't have families, so we're it. Sometimes our presence, a touch, or a look is more helpful than words.

Wise speech is something you can explore for a lifetime. Try for a period of perhaps a day, a week, or longer to play with different forms of wise speech and see what you learn. Here are some ideas: don't criticize anyone; be curious and open-minded about people's motivations; speak kindly to yourself and others; talk about people who are not there as if they were; at the end of the day take stock of all your interactions: Which did you enjoy? Which were meaningful? If you tend to be very quiet, what would it be like to speak more, and if you tend to speak a lot, what would it be like to speak less? When you do these exercises, what do you learn?

Life Changes

Each day, each year, each chapter of our life is marked by continual change. There are transition points in the natural world: dawn, dusk, seasons, the lunar cycle, the migration of birds and animals. There are natural transitions in our lives: the conception of a child, the birth of a child, birthdays, puberty, the menstrual cycle, marriage, anniversaries, divorce, menopause, retirement, aging, and death. These have been marked in different ways throughout history. Around the world different cultures mark them in different ways. They are opportunities for reflection, where stepping back, appreciation, and review can be helpful. One hundred years ago the average life expectancy was less than 50; now it is closer to 80. This means we have more life to live. Many young people might expect to have quite a few different jobs in their lives. Relationships, with siblings, friends, partners, now last significantly longer than they did for our grandparents. A more deliberative period of pausing and asking questions can help you navigate these transition points.

The Ancient Oak: "Wintering"

Winter is a season when trees, plants, and animals seem to hunker down and recede. Trees lose their leaves or bark and seem to be asleep. Animals hibernate beneath the ground, sometimes beneath meters of snow. But while it is easy to imagine there is no life, if you look carefully, you can see that the trees are protecting themselves from the elements, but there are dormant buds waiting for spring, and deep in the roots and trunk of the tree there is a lot of life. The hibernating animals' hearts are beating, and their lungs are breathing, albeit much slowed down, using energy reserves they laid down in autumn.

In the same way, loss, sadness, depression, and illness can be a form of winter, in which we hunker down, conserve our energy, just are, while we wait for the inevitable spring to come. There is a wisdom to wintering.

PRACTICE: **Reflection on Key Transitions Points**

You can follow along on our website.

The Responding Wisely practice can be extended to transitions in our lives, both small (the start and end of a day) and large (career changes). They provide a chance to be and know these moments more fully and from a variety of perspectives. Are you moving through these transitions, guided true north by your values? Maybe this is a chance to reset either your values or what you're doing.

MOHAMMED: *At the Nikah, our wedding day, my father and mother said to me over breakfast, "Today is going to fly by. Let us worry about all the practicalities; you enjoy the day and being with your new wife." I took their advice, and I have so many vivid and rich memories of that day, being surrounded by family and friends, our vows in front of them all, dancing. Some of our friends formed a band and played our favorite music, as well as some traditional music. It really felt like a signing of a contract, surrounded by people we love, followed by a celebration. Every year my wife and I sit down together on our anniversary and renew our vows. We've updated them as kids arrived, as she became successful in her career, as my disability meant I could no longer do sports or indeed any physical work. It helped our marriage evolve through the changes in our lives, as individuals but as a family too. It helps us enjoy each other, but also when we have had difficulties and arguments, there is always a sense of trust and respect. That respect alongside a sense of renewal and evolving has kept our marriage current and vibrant.*

SAM: *It was my day off. When I woke up, I realized I was dead tired from the week, so I turned over and slept a few hours more. When I finally got out of bed I went to the fridge. Empty. So I thought, "Brunch it is." I biked to my favorite café, and as I was sipping my coffee, sitting by my bike, ping. An email comes in from an agency looking for nurses in another country—that sounded exciting, but am I brave enough? Where do I want to live? What kind of job would I enjoy? Do I want to really work at this career or have more of work–home balance, for meeting a partner? I was buzzing about all the possibilities.*

The Ancient Oak: What Am I Becoming?

Tempora mutantur, nos et mutamur in illis. The times change, and we change with them.

If I am changing, what am I in the process of becoming?

We are changing all the time, whether we like it or not. Why not change with awareness and have a say in the changes?

Responding Wisely: A Lifelong Project

It's time to start living the life you imagined.
—HENRY JAMES

Being able to see reactivity with friendliness enables you to step back and create some space. In this space you can choose a response that is aligned with your values. The more you do this, the more naturalized it becomes. This in turn broadens and builds your sense of capacity and trust that you can navigate a whole variety of situations, not only in fair weather but also through storms.

If you get to taste the fruits of this work in everyday life, it becomes something you choose to do because it enriches your life, which you enjoy, rather than something you feel obliged to do. In time it can even become just what you do and who you are. You learn that it is possible to live in ways that have meaning and purpose, that create contentment and joy, not only for you but also for those around you whose lives you touch and for the wider world. Living well is what we'll turn to in the remaining chapters.

10

Cool Head and Warm Heart
The Art of Balance and Equanimity

Icarus was a young man whose talented father, Daedalus, had built them each a set of wings to escape their imprisonment on a Greek island. Daedalus had made the wings out of feathers and fabric, held together by wax, which needed to be soft enough to allow the feathers to flex. Daedalus was worried about Icarus's youthful energy and warned him, "If you fly too close to the sun, the wax will melt. If you fly too close to the sea, the wax will harden. In both cases the wings will fail. Please stay in the middle." Icarus famously flew too close to the sun and came crashing down to earth.

How can we find the middle way that avoids the extremes of too much excitement and change, on the one hand, or too much sluggishness, on the other? How can we enjoy living fully without losing our balance? Balance plays out in every area of our life. How can we enjoy the good moments in our lives without getting overly upset when they end? How can we bear the difficult moments, reminding ourselves that "this too will pass"? Can we love fully, knowing that one day we may lose that person? What makes it possible to invest ourselves in a project, knowing that it may not work out?

Everything we have covered has laid the foundations for balance and equanimity. Stable attention alongside a new way of knowing creates the opportunity to meet any moment with a cool head. Befriending our experience is meeting these moments with a warm heart. Equanimity is an attitude and skill that can be developed.

This chapter outlines how a cool head and warm heart can help you stay balanced in both your inner and outer lives and how you can cultivate balance throughout your life.

Balance in Life

There are so many drivers steering our lives: praise, blame, the endless pursuit of happiness, material wealth; the desire to be liked, to fit in, to have good looks, to stay youthful, to be famous; all the have-to-dos of life. The list is endless. It's no surprise that we're constantly asking, "What do I need more of?" and "What do I want less of?" and thinking "I ought to," "I should," "It's not enough," "I'm not good enough," or "Something is missing." In any moment we're standing in the middle of all of this, trying our best to stay balanced. It can be exhausting.

What does it mean to find balance and equanimity in these moments? It means being fully engaged while keeping our cool. It does not mean being distant from or cut off from life. Rather, it is standing up close to our experiences, whether they're pleasant or unpleasant, staying present without being overwhelmed, with an attitude of friendliness. Moving in close to experience means we see the moment of judgment, impulsivity, or call to action. This applies to both the moment-by-moment unfolding experience and the choices we make in our lives throughout our day and indeed our lives.

> SAM: *Sometimes when the bus is packed, I have to stand, hanging on to one of those overhead straps. It's a simple joy. The bus going along, stopping and starting, turning and bumping. Me standing alongside everyone, all of us holding on to the straps, swaying like trees in the wind.*

Equanimity is closely related to appreciation, which helps us turn toward the good. It is also closely related to care, which helps us turn toward difficulties, in ourselves, others, and the wider world. Our awareness, like the bright and warming sun, shines light on all things equally. This is the basis for finding ease, contentment, peace, and connection in our lives. It is an intention, an attitude, and it can be cultivated.

The Barefoot Professor: Balance

Our sense of physical balance is our brain working together with the input of several sensory systems, our eyes (visual system), our inner ears (vestibular system), and our spatial awareness (proprioception). Losing our sense of balance can create dizziness, vertigo, even nausea. Our sense of mental balance is also the result of various brain and body systems working together. Losing our sense of mental balance is just as discombobulating, creating unease and anxiety.

Cultivating Balance and Equanimity

How can you cultivate a cool head and a warm heart? How can you stay balanced with everything that tries to pull you off balance? You have already put many of the conditions for equanimity in place. Paying attention is a good start. An attitude of curiosity helps you welcome whatever you see as it is, without elaboration. Standing back and asking, "What is this?" helps you take a wider perspective. Meeting all these moments with friendliness expands our capacity for steadiness and balance. Recognizing, allowing, and savoring pleasant experiences guards against sentimentality and develops an appreciation that is deeper and more real. Recognizing, allowing, and meeting unpleasant experiences, the first arrow, with attitudes of friendliness, interest, courage, and care, means they do not escalate into suffering with a volley of "second arrows" (which we covered in Chapters 5 and 6).

Equanimity can be cultivated through mindfulness practice, but it takes time. The mindfulness practices are exactly that, *practice,* so that when pain, pleasure, or your desires overwhelm you, you can draw on what you've learned and find balance.

Equanimity in Mindfulness Practices

All the mindfulness practices, such as awareness of your mind and body (Chapter 3) and cultivation of attitudes (Chapter 7), offer a chance to develop equanimity. This can be in the moment you first become aware of sensations, feelings, impulses, and thoughts or at any point in the chain of your unfolding moment-to-moment experience. The earlier in the process you can recognize and bring awareness to the tendency to label your experiences as pleasant/unpleasant and like/not like, the more likely you are to be able to create a space in which you can respond and not react. Equanimity is keeping a cool head and warm heart in these moments.

Cultivating Balance in Our Bodies

Mindfulness of the body is a lifetime practice. Scanning your body means that you encounter the full range of bodily sensations—energy, agitation, calm, sleepiness, the many sensations you label "pain," sensual pleasure in all its many forms. The Body Scan teaches you to move your attention through the body without highlighting any one area of the body, or preferring any one sensation, over others (to remind yourself about the Body Scan, see Chapter 2, page 37). This is where you learn to step out of your natural tendency to pay attention to difficulties, to like pleasant moments and pass over pretty well everything else. This is a powerful lesson for our lives. Our preferences and labeling of experience are so automatic. You're learning to step out of the automatic "turning away from" or "turning toward" things you don't and do like. And you learn that it is not what's happening in your body that knocks you off balance, but your reactions.

> SAM: *When I first started doing Body Scans, I hit a wall of resistance and impatience. The itchiness, the wanting to get up and do something else, anything else, wanting oblivion, sleep. It was tough to face—I wasn't exactly thrilled with what surfaced. It took weeks before I could see that my impatience was like a curtain veiling a whole production inside my body. What I feared most was mostly in my imagination. Sure, my body has some itchiness; some urges, definitely; some agitation, yes. Sure, I can own up to being a bit of a thrill seeker. But in all of it, I learned I could stay with, even learn from it. The agitation had a lot to do with what I hadn't processed from my day. The itchiness was bearable and pointed to a need to use the ointment I know helps.*

Cultivating a Balanced Mind

Bringing awareness to thoughts, moods, and emotions is a chance to practice equanimity for whatever you find. Can you find a way to stay balanced toward gain and loss, fame and shame, praise and blame, happiness and misery? Awareness imbued with friendliness helps you recognize a mood as a mood, a thought as a mental event, an emotion as an emotion, and an impulse as an impulse. This helps us dismantle the house of cards we've constructed about what it takes to be happy in terms of achievements, fame, and praise. Without this house of cards, we're freer to meet our experiences and ourselves with appreciation and care.

When you extend this quality of friendly awareness to the ever-changing patterns of your mind, you see that moods and thoughts last longer when you react to them with liking and not liking. When you give up preferences—"I like this, I don't like this"—sensations, moods, thoughts, and impulses arise and fall away, arise and fall away. Stillness emerges, suffering softens, joy grows.

> LING: *It takes a lot not to be scared of and smashed by my wrecking-ball thoughts. But recognizing them and standing back was a great start. Trying to stay steady when I can sense their power is good progress for me.*

Cultivating Balance in Real Life, for Life

The place where we're looking to develop equanimity is in our day-to-day lives. Each day will present its share of hassles. Changes in your health are inevitable, other people don't always act the way you want them to, and your life doesn't always run as you expected. There are serious challenges in the world's changing climate, geopolitics, pandemics, and migration. Equanimity helps you stay steady in your life, with all its unpredictability and uncertainty, without getting carried away or lost.

> SOPHIA: *I recently gave Noah, my grandson, some weebles that I'd found packed away in the attic. Weebles are these old-fashioned wooden toy characters shaped like an egg that find their way upright even if you knock them over. They belonged to his mum when she was a child, and we'd had had this expression in our family from the ads, "Weebles wobble, but they don't fall down." Anytime someone had a wobble, this was our family's way of saying, "It's okay, you've had a wobble, but you'll be okay."*

The Ancient Oak: Equanimity and Serenity

We're developing the serenity to accept the things we cannot change, the courage to change the things we can, and the wisdom to know the difference. Serenity needs a cool head and a warm heart, courage involves embracing what we like, bearing what we don't, being okay with change, and having the courage to make necessary changes. Wisdom involves tapping into our different ways of knowing and making discerning choices with a sense of trust.

This central idea, sometimes called the *serenity prayer*, has its roots in many philosophical (for example, stoicism) and religious traditions (for example, the Bhagavad Gita in Hinduism and the Four Noble Truths in Buddhism) and is widely used in mainstream 12-step recovery groups.

> SOPHIA: *When I was first diagnosed with Parkinson's, I got busy, compulsively so. I researched it, got second opinions, changed my diet, bought a fitness tracker, and joined different support groups. I guess I was hoping that somewhere I'd find the key to unlocking this awful place I found myself, a good life but an awful diagnosis. The busyness was driven by worry, resentment, "Why me?" and sometimes outright terror. Parkinson's disease <u>demands</u> equanimity; I had to accept that its progression was inevitable. I knew people who had had it, and now I'm seeing it for myself.*
>
> *One evening I was on a sand bank with my daughter and grandson. The sun was starting to set, and the tide was coming in; we'd have to move in an hour or two as the*

sea would reclaim the whole sand bank. Noah and I had spent the afternoon build-
ing sandcastles, and now I was reading a self-help book about living with Parkinson's.
Noah came to sit on my lap, sucking his thumb. He fell asleep as the sun set and the
heat went out of the day. I felt so much happiness and love in those moments. I realized
that my struggle to come to terms with my diagnosis was feeding my fear. Carrying
Noah back to the car, I put the self-help book in the bin and chatted to my daughter
about what we'd cook for dinner.

The Parkinson's was just as inevitable and powerful as the tide. I started to intro-
duce these phrases into my daily meditation:

"I care for you deeply; things are as they are. I'll take joy in all that is right with
my body and life. I accept, allow, and embrace, as best I can, all that is weakening in
my body." I'd end my daily mindfulness practice with a sense of purpose to carry these
intentions into my day and live each day fully.

I had a powerful sense that, like the sandcastle, everything is impermanent, and
that really supports my equanimity—"This too will pass." More and more I was able
to live this in my day-to-day life.

Children love to build sandcastles on a beach. And we know that the tide
will inevitably come in and wash them away, returning the sand and the shells
to the sea. The building and washing away are all moments that we can choose
to be present for— with all the attitudes that are part of befriending our minds
and our lives, interest, appreciation, care, and letting go, awake to both the
appreciation and the loss, with equanimity.

What do you learn when you're able to do this? It reinforces what you've
learned so far, that the links in the chains of reactivity in your thinking and
behavior can be broken. That the earlier in the chain of reactivity you can
recognize the point at which you lose your poise and balance, the less likely
you are to be carried away by it. The earlier in a chain of reactivity that you
can recognize the development of distress and suffering, the easier it is to break
the links of the chain. In time, you can short-circuit reactivity altogether. If
you can recognize sensations, moods, impulses, or thoughts that are pleasant
or wholesome, you can cultivate these into contentment, ease, connection, joy,
and love. These moments can become actions aligned with your values that
support your well-being and the well-being of others.

MOHAMMED: *After my back injury, my body became a battlefield. I was struggling*
with pain, putting on weight, not being able to do all the things I used to do. All those
years of training and becoming the best athlete, up in flames. I'd resist it, pretending
it wasn't happening. Then when that didn't work, I catastrophized. It took me to some
dark places: "If my life is going to be like this, then I don't want to be alive."

It took years, but I have reclaimed my body. What's helped? My wife's support, my faith, realizing I am a good dad and husband, getting into following sports, the mindfulness practice, especially the mindful movement. When I was an athlete, I had to relate to my body as something to train to the nth degree, year in, year out. I used to work with my sports coaches, but now I work with my Iman. He helped me see that my body is a gift from God, a gift that I can honor.

The Three-Step Breathing Space

The Breathing Space is a great place to develop equanimity. It bridges from mindfulness practice to your everyday life.

The Barefoot Professor:
Affect in the Breathing Space

Psychologists use the word *affect* to describe our general sense of how we are doing. While it is a bit of a simplification, we can say it has two key dimensions:

1. Our level of *arousal*, on a dimension from totally calm to highly stimulated (excited, agitated)
2. *Valence*, on a dimension from pleasant to unpleasant

In her 2017 book *How Emotions Are Made*, Professor Lisa Feldman Barrett suggests we can take these two dimensions and create four poles. High arousal and pleasant might be elated (maybe how we feel at the birth of a healthy child); low arousal and unpleasant might be depressed. Every other state can be mapped somewhere on these two dimensions. The key point is that we can in any moment note our general sense of how we're doing in terms of arousal and valence, our affect.

How can the Breathing Space be fine-tuned to build equanimity? The first way is by learning to note in Step 1 your sense of how you're doing, your affect, in terms of arousal and pleasantness/unpleasantness. The possible flavors of this moment are endless—upset, content, grateful, pleased, lethargic, calm. This noting is important because it has implications for Step 2 and Step 3.

In Step 2, you can choose an anchor that fits the state of mind and body that revealed itself in Step 1. More than likely you have a go-to general-purpose anchor. For many people this is their breath. But as you've been discovering, you'll need some other anchors for when you're in different places on these dimensions. When you're aroused, and potentially around something difficult (fear, for example), you'll need a sturdier anchor. When you're feeling flat, you'll need an anchor that is easier to attend to and that maybe even ups your level of energy.

In Step 3, having noted how you're doing and then anchored yourself, you can build equanimity by tailoring your response. Can you turn toward the pleasant with a sense of appreciation, savoring, gratitude, and joy? Can you learn to turn toward the neutral by dialing up your sense of curiosity and patience? Can you learn to turn toward the unpleasant with kindness, care, and courage? Can you tune in to your level of arousal and respond wisely?

Like all the attitudes of mindfulness, equanimity can also be cultivated directly.

PRACTICE: **Contentment**

You can follow along on our website.

In this practice you steady and anchor yourself in the usual way. When you feel anchored and steady, ask some questions to support cultivating contentment: "Is anything lacking *in this moment*? What else, in this moment, right now, is needed to feel a sense of ease and peace?" The real teaching here comes when you stay very close to this moment. If you notice your mind wandering, you start judging, or wider questions about your life come up, escorting your attention back to *this moment*. "What else, right now, is needed to feel a sense of ease and peace?" What you're exploring is what it means to rest in this moment, exactly as it is, without trying to change or fix it, with ease. Can you rest in the small space between the ending of the outbreath and the beginning of the next breath, to rest in the quiet between sounds, to rest in the body?

This can be a powerful practice in cultivating a sense of things as they are, of *coming to rest* in any given moment. If only you can open fully to this moment, exactly as it is, you may find that there is a real sense of contentment and ease. For many people the question "What else, in this moment, do I need to feel a sense of ease?"—even when their lives are full or challenging—can be very steadying. For some people the thinking mind kicks in with wider questions of what might be missing in our lives or the world. The Vietnamese mindfulness teacher Thich Nhat Hahn said, "Peace is one breath away." What he means is that whatever is happening in our lives or even in the world, our breath and body are always available to us as a refuge, somewhere to find peace amid whatever else is happening.

The Ancient Oak: Finding Peace in Any Moment

Rudyard Kipling's "If" is a poem that in many ways is about equanimity.

> If you can keep your head when all about you
> Are losing theirs and blaming it on you,
> If you can trust yourself when all men doubt you,
> But make allowance for their doubting too;
> If you can wait and not be tired by waiting,
> Or being lied about, don't deal in lies,
> Or being hated, don't give way to hating,
> And yet don't look too good, nor talk too wise:
> If you can dream—and not make dreams your master;
> If you can think—and not make thoughts your aim;
> If you can meet with Triumph and Disaster
> And treat those two impostors just the same;
> If you can bear to hear the truth you've spoken
> Twisted by knaves to make a trap for fools,
> Or watch the things you gave your life to, broken,
> And stoop and build 'em up with worn-out tools:
> If you can make one heap of all your winnings
> And risk it on one turn of pitch-and-toss,
> And lose, and start again at your beginnings
> And never breathe a word about your loss;
> If you can force your heart and nerve and sinew
> To serve your turn long after they are gone,
> And so hold on when there is nothing in you
> Except the Will which says to them: 'Hold on!'
> If you can talk with crowds and keep your virtue,
> Or walk with Kings—nor lose the common touch,
> If neither foes nor loving friends can hurt you,
> If all men count with you, but none too much;
> If you can fill the unforgiving minute
> With sixty seconds' worth of distance run,
> Yours is the Earth and everything that's in it,
> And—which is more—you'll be a Man, my son!

Kipling is inviting you to "keep your head" when everyone else is not, when people doubt or turn against you, when things go well or badly. It is one of the most popular poems of all time, perhaps because it speaks directly to the reader about staying balanced in the midst of the many things that can knock us off balance.

Mindfulness practice is in many ways about internalizing these ideas. Namely, that balance is available with us, and it is possible to restore balance even in the most challenging situations.

SAM: *Through my mindfulness practice and just everyday life I've learned to smile at myself. I am a bit all or nothing and I'm okay with that; it is me. Always been a thrill seeker. Back in the day I climbed trees and rode my bike too fast. Thankfully, the worst that happened is I once fell out of a tree and broke my arm. When I came out, for a while I was all about random hookups; sometimes what I was doing was on the edge. But by going to too far, I've figured out where my boundaries are. Kayaking is my thing now, especially whitewater. Last week there was a lot of rain, and I knew a river that was going to be wild. So, I went out on the river on Saturday. As I was kayaking, the river banks ripped past. I was loving every moment. Then I got to a big weir on the left—too crazy to go down—and a bridge to the right, water coursing through the three arches like a beast. In that split second I had to choose a track—weir or one of three bridge arches. There was no way to go back, and it was too late to track to the bank. I went for the bridge arch on the right and said to myself under my breath, over and over, "Trust the river." In those heart-pounding moments I felt extraordinary aliveness, mixed with peace, and, yeah, adrenaline was in the mix too. (Smiling) Lived to tell the tale.*

The Ancient Oak: A Traditional Chinese Story, Originally Based on Tao's Teaching

Once upon a time, there was a hard-working farmer in the central region of China. He was married and had one teenage son who also worked on the farm. He didn't have a lot of money, and, instead of a tractor, he had a horse that he'd taken care of for many years to plough the fields on the family farm. The horse was now old and struggling with the work. One afternoon, while working in the fields, the horse's heart failed, and he died suddenly. The family was very sorry to lose their horse after years of service but did not have enough money to buy another. Everyone in the village said, "Oh, what a horrible thing to happen. How difficult for the farmer and his family." *(Pause)*

The farmer said, "Maybe, maybe not."

He was so calm that everyone in the village got together and gave him a new horse as a gift. The farmer took good care of the new horse, to settle it into its life on the farm. But a couple days later, the new horse jumped the fence and ran away. Everyone in the village shook their heads and said, "What a poor fellow!"

The farmer said, "Maybe, maybe not."

Eventually, the horse found his way home, and everyone again said, "That's lucky, the farmer has his horse back."

The farmer said, "Maybe, maybe not."

Later in the year, the farmer's son went out riding on the horse and fell and broke his leg. Everyone in the village said, "What a shame for the poor boy."

The farmer said, "Maybe, maybe not."

Two days later, the army came into the village to draft new recruits. When they saw that the farmer's son had a broken leg, they decided not to recruit him.

Everyone said, "What a fortunate young man."

The farmer said, "Maybe, maybe not."

In Taoism the story points to the fact that good fortune can sometimes follow disaster, and equally disaster can follow good fortune. It teaches us equanimity.

TROUBLESHOOTING: Balance: What It Is and Isn't, What's Helpful and What Isn't

Equanimity is often misunderstood as being detached, resigned, or passive. But it is none of these things. Instead, it is being fully engaged, but with a cool head and warm heart. It is learning to kayak, rather than resist the current. It is being fully present with the myriad facets of our lives, good, bad, or indifferent, with wholehearted responsiveness that aligns with our values and supports our well-being and the well-being of others.

Equanimity applies to many dimensions, where the lines between what is helpful and unhelpful can be vanishingly thin. Here are just a few:

- Timorous–bold
- Authentic–selfish
- Strong–vulnerable
- Open–closed
- Trusting–mistrustful
- Foolhardy–courageous

What you're learning is where the balance lies for you, in different situations and at different times.

Taking It Further: Learning to Stay Balanced in an Uncertain, Changing, and Complex World

Equanimity can be practiced in the tiny moments in your day, your relationships, and many of the pressing issues in the wider world.

> SAM: *When the Covid pandemic hit, it was madness. Patients were really sick, but no one knew what coronavirus was or how to treat it. The consultant and senior nurse ran the ICU with incredible professionalism and icy calm. But all of the training in the world could not have prepared us for some of the shifts. Their leadership, our positive team culture, and our training were our lifelines through some incredibly difficult situations and months. I am not going to sugar-coat it; we saw some terrible situations. But the team culture was solid; we had each other's backs, helping everyone stay afloat and process the craziness we were witnessing. It was a wild ride those months.*

Cultivating equanimity helps you stay balanced when things happen that could easily throw you off balance. This might be close to home, someone saying something that makes you angry, for example, or unsettling events in the world, like the Covid pandemic. Fortunately, there are some mindfulness practices that develop equanimity. Remember, this is mindfulness in real life, *for* life, so it may be that at different times and phases in your life these practices will be more or less helpful to you. Trust your intuition, but when you make a commitment to a practice, make the commitment for a period of days, months, or even years. Revisiting the comparison with gardening, it takes a long time to develop a mature garden. Landscaping the mind similarly takes persistence, patience, and time.

PRACTICE: Letting Go

You can follow along on our website.

This practice is intended to cultivate equanimity by exploring what happens when you let go. Start by scanning your body with a sense of openness. Is there a sense of ease? If you find areas of contraction or tension, try as best you can to let go of the tension. If it helps, use your outbreath to have a sense of letting go.

Find an anchor and steady your mind. Take as long as you need and know this anchor is somewhere you can come back to at any point.

Next open your awareness, so that there is a sense of allowing whatever comes up to be welcome. Move up close, allow experiences to be as they are, with an attitude of befriending whatever you find. Let go of any need to fix or change anything.

If it feels helpful, here are some words you might say to yourself:

"Letting go of my need for control and certainty."

Continue with this phrase for as long as it feels helpful.

Allow your experience to be as it is; you're not trying to fix or change anything.

This practice is intended to incline the mind to equanimity by welcoming and accepting whatever comes up and letting go of our need to control and be okay. The closer this can be to the point where you start striving for what you like and rejecting what you don't, the more you learn to nip reactivity in the bud.

You can adapt the phrase to whatever you may be struggling with in your life. For example, often it is other people and relationships. You might play with phrases like "Letting go of my need for love and care." The phrases are intended to speak directly to what drives reactivity. Naturally, we need to have a sense of control and be loved. But can you find a way of living without being relentlessly driven by them and without being too unsettled when inevitably things don't go the way you want, and people don't act the way you'd like them to?

PRACTICE: The Tree Revisited

You can follow along on our website.

I introduced the tree practice in Chapter 8 (page 156). As well as perspective, it develops equanimity. Trees face the different cycles of night and day, seasons, and weather—they seed, germinate, mature, and eventually die. They have to adapt, as the weather and seasons change and as they mature and grow. Recently, we've learned they can communicate with one another through their root systems and foliage. Different trees do this in different ways—pine, orange, oak, coconut, willow, chestnut. . . . In a spirit of openness and playfulness, use the tree practice to cultivate equanimity, including amid all the changes in your life. In your practice, bring to mind a tree that has that sense of steadiness through change and imagine yourself as that tree. See how the tree can help you stay steady and balanced in your mindfulness practice and then throughout your day.

PRACTICE: The 50–50 Practice Revisited

When are you most likely to be unbalanced? It is relatively easy to stay balanced if you are on your own and have control over your environment. The hard work comes when you're with other people, especially when there are conflict, competition, differences in expectations, or situations that push you to react in extreme ways. Our values are different and inevitably rub up against one another. The 50–50 practice (Chapter 3, page 65) is about splitting your awareness between what is happening in the situation and what is happening for you. Here the 50–50 practice is first a barometer of how you are in the situation. But then, by anchoring part of your awareness in your body, it also serves to keep you steady, providing the space to respond wisely.

SOPHIA: *At schoolteacher–parent conferences we're always full-on, and later in my career more so because parents seemed to have higher expectations of their children, the school, and so became more demanding. It felt like a minefield, sometimes, and if I am honest there were certain parents I dreaded seeing. I started using the 50–50 practice in the moments between meetings.*

I remember this one boy: he was a playground bully, and his dad, who I had never met before, came with him. When I saw his dad, for the first time I had real empathy for the boy. His father swaggered across the room in a threatening way, sat down, and demanded to know why his son wasn't doing better. His son, who normally swaggered around the school, seemed cowed next to him. I had this sense of myself being like an oak, rooted, strong, able to weather anything. As this swaggering, combative dad spoke, I felt present and steady, which helped me listen calmly. At one point I caught the boy's eye, and we smiled at each other with an understanding I don't remember having before.

We're exposed to many polarized debates about important issues—politics, reproductive and abortion rights, criminal justice, asylum, immigration, gender identity, religion, inequalities in all sorts of areas, and end-of-life care. When we take extreme positions, we can be so sure that we are right. From this position it is much easier to put down or attack anyone who doesn't agree with us. History teaches us that when people take this to extremes, it leads to conflict between groups of people, wars, and even genocide. What does this have to do with equanimity? These are examples of groups of people, nations, even whole groups of people losing perspective and balance. But groups are made up of a collection of individuals. We all play our part in polarization and its effects. Keeping our balance means being able to see and challenge polarization and extremism. When Simone Weil said that "attention is the rarest and purest form of generosity," what she meant was that it enables us to remind ourselves of our values when we're distracted, or worse, coerced. When we do this, we have at least a chance to find ways to ask, "Is what I am doing here helpful?" As we saw in Chapter 9, this helps us respond wisely, in this case toward solutions that are constructive and, where possible, a win for everyone.

SAM: *I wrote my dissertation about euthanasia. I did a deep dive into the books and talked to people on both sides—pro- and anti-euthanasia. I honestly didn't have a clear view when I started out, and mostly I still don't. But here is what I learned. Both groups had good reasons for why they held the views they did. But what hit me hard was that both sides weren't really prepared to really listen to each other, they were so sure of themselves. I remember thinking if only they really listen to each other, they might not change their point of view, but they'd crack open the door to better possibilities for the people at the end of their lives.*

Balance as an Anchor throughout Life

As we saw with Icarus finding a middle way between the hot sun and the cold sea, finding balance can anchor us and safeguard us against extremes. The heat can have a very powerful pull on us. The cool air in the middle may not seem that appealing. But equanimity is about leaning into the hot, cold, and cool; the pleasant, the unpleasant, and the neutral. In a sense appreciation of what is good in our lives and care toward what is difficult are the same—they are moments that require recognition, letting be, patience, and trust.

SOPHIA: *Make hay while the sun shines. Make love while it rains.*

As you learn to develop a sense of equanimity, you learn to engage with every aspect of your life with awareness, care, and compassion. You can learn to live fully and wholeheartedly, something we turn to in the next chapter.

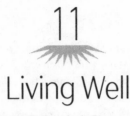

11

Living Well

Taking Care of Ourselves,
Our Relationships, and the World

Everything has been figured out, except how to live.
—JEAN-PAUL SARTRE

What can we do to live well and to flourish? What do we know about what supports our well-being? How can we live in a way that sustains not just us but our communities and the wider world? These are questions that contemplative traditions, philosophy, the arts, and many scientific disciplines including psychology help us answer. Our physical needs, security, and relationships are the foundation of our survival. But they are not all we need; they are what we build on. To live well, we also need what is meaningful and gives us a sense of accomplishment, whether it's work or sports, studies, family, friends, fun, sexuality, or just time out relaxing. What feels meaningful to us often lines up with our values. Finally, to live well means living sustainably, taking care of others and the world, because without that we have no community or place to live in. This chapter pulls together and builds on all the learning so far to reflect on what it means to live well and sustainably.

Living Well, Living Sustainably

In the same way you "practice" any skill, you can practice the skills that support your well-being.

SOPHIA: *Yesterday was a long day. I started the day quickly walking Rufus, before bundling him in the car to take care of Noah because it was a school snow day, and my daughter didn't want to let down her clients in her acupuncture practice. Noah is fun, but full on, and I had the whole day with him mostly indoors because of the snow. When my daughter got back at 7:00, I needed to make a trip to the supermarket, before going home, getting something to eat, and then collapsing on the sofa to watch an hour of mindless TV. I fell asleep on the sofa with a sense that I'd survived a very full day, grateful to fall asleep. But I also wondered if this is sustainable given my health; my Parkinson's is fortunately still in the early stages, mild, and seems to be the slow progression type, at least for now, but I have to take care of myself.*

Too often we pay attention to self-care only when we're forced to, when we're already in dire straits. This is a bit like rescuing an exhausted kayaker out of the river, in perilous danger close to Niagara Falls, or worse still, badly battered and needing to be rescued at the bottom of Niagara Falls. So, living well means learning and applying well-being skills, pacing ourselves, learning from experience, taking care along the way, and knowing and working within our limits. More than all this, taking care means equipping ourselves so that we can live with a sense of security, with direction, and enjoy the journey. Kayak lessons start on dry land and then progress to a swimming pool, and only then in manageable steps to more and more challenging outdoor waterways. Over time, kayakers who have learned these skills, including knowing their limits, can navigate white water if they choose to.

Skills that build well-being are a necessary foundation for living well over a lifetime. Once you have these, you can add skills for when things go wrong, which inevitably they do. Finally, you need some skills for those inevitable transitions and passages in life, including times when you end up in dire straits.

Mindfulness Practices for Protecting and Building Well-Being

All the mindfulness practices I've introduced so far are ways of learning about and cultivating our minds and bodies. This is a form of self-care. As we've already discussed at length in Chapter 3, when you learn to tune in to your body, like a readout from a modern car, it tells us all sorts of helpful things. Are you energized or tired? Are you holding tension, and if so, where? Is there a sense of ease or pleasure, and if so, where? Are you dehydrated or hungry? Is there a need to connect?

How can the attitudes of mindfulness (Chapter 7) help you live well? In any moment or situation, you can ask yourself "What is the state of my mind right now?" Is it curious or closed, open-hearted or judgmental, energized or lethargic? You can dial particular attitudes up or down. If you find you've become judgmental, perhaps you need more kindness and equanimity.

If you notice physical or emotional pain, perhaps you need care. You can recognize and then intentionally reset your attitude of mind. It is worth reminding yourself of appreciation in particular, as appreciation is an attitude that has far-reaching effects. It has a way of opening up, broadening, and making everything seem more possible.

PRACTICE: Open Awareness

You can follow along on our website.

This is a practice for developing awareness and a sense of space. It starts in the usual way, with making any adjustments to your posture and taking a moment to steady. Then when you feel steady, sweep your awareness through your body—the base, the trunk, your limbs, your head—with a sense of space in and around your body.

Having opened your awareness to body sensations, the next step is opening up your awareness to whatever is present. This has a quality of zooming out, so that any sensations, sounds, moods, impulses, thoughts, or images are noticed, seen, and allowed to be exactly as they are, experiences coming and going. This includes mind wandering as something your mind does, but at the moment you become aware of it, broaden out again to awareness of moment-by-moment experiences coming and going.

It can help to have a sense of yourself like a tree. The tree can sway and adapt but remains rooted and majestic as all these experiences, like weather systems, birds, animals, and people, come and go.

As you bring this practice to a close, make a commitment to reconnecting with this sense of steadiness, balance, and space throughout your day.

Many people describe finding stillness and peace in this practice, as their experiences are seen with interest, friendliness, and care for what they are, moment by moment. Rather than choosing to anchor or foreground something in awareness, you open awareness up and see what is there, allowing it to be in the floodlight. This requires having first learned to stabilize your attention, so that from this stable foundation you can open out to broader awareness. Here you're able to allow and hold whatever is around in awareness, the unfolding, continual stream of whatever is present—sensations, moods, impulses, thoughts, sounds, perhaps even several of these in parallel, or moving in and out of awareness. Awareness is like the whole sky, where everything in the realm of our senses, our body and mind, is potentially in awareness. This is hard to explain; the best way to understand is to, when you feel ready, try the practice for yourself at a time you feel in a steady enough place to do it. Don't rush it, though; this is quite an advanced practice that needs good foundations in place and learning through practice.

Taking Care of Ourselves

What keeps you going, nourishes you, depletes you, is important to you? It can help to take an inventory.

Taking an Inventory of Your Needs

The hierarchy of needs plays out here. Do you feel safe in your day-to-day life? If not, this is a priority and needs to be addressed. It is a basic human right to live in safety and security. Are you prioritizing basic physical self-care—sleep, hydration, healthy food, and exercise? These are all areas that can make real and immediate differences to your well-being. Health and leisure centers, family doctors, nurse practitioners, apps, and many online resources can provide information and advice. (See our Mindfulness for Life website for more resources.)

> ### EXERCISE: What Does Taking Care Look Like for You?
>
> *You can follow along on our website.*
>
> These essential foundations of well-being can be built on to create conditions for well-being.
>
> From a typical day last week, write out how you spent your time. Chunk the day into the main segments. For example, got out of bed, had a cup of coffee or tea, had a shower, breakfast, caught the bus to college, had a walk at lunchtime with a friend . . . all the way to the end of the day.
>
> Now go through the list and next to each activity ask, "Did this nourish me?" If it did, put an arrow pointing up next to it: ↑. Now ask, "Did any of the activities drain me or deplete me?" If they did, put an arrow pointing down next to them: ↓. Some may be neutral, neither nourishing nor depleting you; that's fine—just leave them as they are. Some may sometimes lift you up and sometimes drain you; here put an upward and downward arrow: ↑↓.
>
> To fill out the list further, maybe scan back over the last few weeks, months, even years. Ask yourself what else nourishes and depletes you, perhaps a change of scene, visiting someone you care about, or a holiday.
>
> This will create a list of what nourishes you and what depletes you. What about things that can be either nourishing or depleting. Here the question is, "What makes the difference?" Taking care of ourselves includes building into our lives ways of nourishing ourselves with activities that you've come to know as pleasurable and rewarding. This is what it means to live well and sustainably, to take an active role in your well-being.

LING: *If I have a good night's sleep, I feel so much better, like my brain has rested and processed stuff while I was asleep, which of course it has. Sleep probably makes the biggest difference between a bad and good day to me.*

SOPHIA: *What nourishes me: nature, swimming, singing, Rufus, my dog, healthy food—and rest. I am lucky to be more or less retired, so I choose a lot of what I do. But I was surprised that spending time with family and friends could be both nourishing and depleting. I need time on my own to recharge my batteries. Also, my grandson can be quite draining, but also nourishing; he is a toddler and has so much energy. Then I realized, to my surprise, that one of my best friends is almost always draining. I feel guilty even having that thought; I need to think about that.*

SAM: *I don't have a car, can't afford it, plus there's nowhere to park. So I cycle to work, and it takes about 20 minutes. Now here's the weird part: weekend bike rides— pure fun. Cycling to work—a chore. That's what I thought until I stopped to look at it—"That doesn't make sense." I switched it up. Dodging traffic on my bike, getting my heart revving first thing; it's a natural wake-up call. And get this: part of my route is through a park. People say it's sketchy with kids doing their thing and smoking dope and there are some people selling drugs. But I roll through it anyway. When I head home, some of the kids throw a "hi" my way, it's like they've found somewhere they feel safe.*

Using Your Inventory to Make Changes in Your Life

Once you have an inventory, you can, as Sam did with cycling to work, ask if some of what nourishes and depletes you can be adjusted. You can make it more of a habit to open your eyes, literally and figuratively, to all that is good in your life, including the many blessings that get overlooked. Savoring and appreciating the good moments more fully, especially when you feel them in your body, turns them into good experiences. It can also extend to doing what is meaningful and aligned with your values. Together this creates the conditions for well-being.

MOHAMMED: *My days are so full—I am exhausted at the end of the day. I have to pray last thing. If I am honest, I'd come to resent having to pray when I am so tired. But I realized from this exercise that prayer is one of the most nourishing parts of my day, so during this last prayer of the day I take the time to appreciate all the blessings of Allah—that changes it into a good ending to my day.*

The Barefoot Professor:
What Happens When We Don't Take Care of Ourselves

When we work too hard, or burn the candle at both ends, we can get run down. We feel tired and flat all the time. When this happens at work, in extremis it is described as burnout. Professor Christina Maslach studied burnout and heard how people described a very particular array of symptoms, including emotional exhaustion, depersonalization, and cynicism. Professor Marie Åsberg studied how this comes about and coined the phrase "exhaustion funnel." It is like traveling down a funnel that gets ever narrower and darker. As people start to get tired, their sense of their ability to cope diminishes, their actual experience of positive and rewarding events reduces, they feel their lives are joyless—until they find themselves at the bottom of the funnel, exhausted.

Taking Care When Things Go Wrong

Everything you have covered so far is about building well-being, which is a way of preventing burnout. Professor Jon Kabat-Zinn suggested a metaphor of "weaving your parachute," so that when you need it, it is there for you. So that when you find that you're not doing well, you know what to do.

MOHAMMED: *My young kids are forever asking questions, and I used to feel my job was to teach them. But really my kids teach me as much as I teach them. For example, when the youngest is tired, she gets irritable and then conks out and sleeps. I just get irritable and then more irritable, and sometimes only later do I realize how tired I am. They can see when this is happening and sometimes will say, "Dad, you need a nap." I occasionally, if I can, have a nap at the same time as my kids now. Go figure.*

The other day I was in a café, and both of my kids were cranky. One was crying, and someone said, trying to be nice, "Can I help?" I was full of shame and rage. But I dealt with it, we went outside, and the one who was crying loves holding my hand. So we held hands as we walked home. When we got home, I cooked some simple food that I know they like, they had a bath, and we read a story. They fell asleep without fuss. That moment in the café was like being in a sandstorm, but my kids teach me that family is also about those moments and riding out the sandstorm.

It can be helpful to have a scale, a bit like the battery icon on your phone: 80–100% means you are doing well, 50% is okay, 70% is good, 20% is low, and below 5% is critical. Different power levels may call for different strategies. At less than 20% phones may enter into "low battery mode," preserving energy. Critical means the phone will soon shut down and need recharging before you can use it again. Obviously, it is best not to get to this point, but if you do, what works for you? Rest, of course, in the form of downtime or sleep. What else works for you? Taking an inventory enables you to build on your list of nourishing activities, adding in what works at these lower battery levels.

> **PRACTICE:**   **Extending Your Self-Care Plan to Respond When Things Have Gone Wrong**
>
> *You can follow along on our website.*
>
> As with all the practices, you start with settling your mind and body, gathering and anchoring your awareness. When you are ready, bring a friend to mind, someone you really trust. Feel their presence—in this moment you are the center of their attention. They have your back. They want the best for you. Ask them, "When I am struggling, what helps, what do I need, what can I do that will get me back on track?" Don't force anything; just see what comes up.

SOPHIA: *My Parkinson's means my battery now never really gets above 70%, but if I take care I can still live my life. I have red lines around exercise, rest, and diet. I do something vigorous every day even though I don't want to; it helps with my Parkinson's symptoms. I take a nap after lunch, which recharges my battery for the rest of the day. I eat well throughout the day because I feel better when I do. After that I think of it as layers of an onion—no pun intended, but every year I get older, I am more comfortable in my own skin. Outer layers of the onion for me are connections with people I love and who love me too, my work. You know, the older I get the more layers there are. I don't care so much what others think, but I know what is important to me.*

Taking It Further:
Living with Joy, Meaning, and Ease

Living well involves more than just taking care of yourself as a daily routine and as part of preparing for challenges and changes. Living well is a lifetime endeavor. The poet Rilke described living well as a life lived in ever-increasing circles that reach out across the world. When you're taking an inventory of what nourishes and drains you, you need to explore how you can live with joy, meaning, and ease. Exploring is endlessly fascinating in and of itself, but you also need to keep it up because what nourishes and depletes you changes as you change and as the world around you changes. Here are some things I have heard people say they have found gives them joy, meaning, and ease:

- "My morning ritual involves a glass of grapefruit juice. My father started every day with a grapefruit. This daily glass of juice reminds me of him, and I feel grateful for all he did for me."
- "I am a social animal; I love going out, parties, weddings—I get charged up by being around people."
- "A group of us meet to walk our dogs. It is not always the same people, but there is always someone to walk with and talk to about everything and nothing."
- "I have notebooks, always have. I carry my notebook with me. Every day I write or sketch in it, without censoring myself—whatever I want."
- "A vigorous walk every day. Fast enough to get my heart going and clear my head."
- "I follow this woman on social media. I love her take on life. She makes me smile every day. Sometimes I even laugh out loud."
- "On my days off, a lazy coffee and my favorite breakfast to start the day."
- "Sunday mornings my partner and I like to make love, nowhere to be, no rush, just us connecting. Bliss."
- "In the evening, watching TV and stroking my cat."
- "My bed is my safe place. I love the feeling of settling down to sleep and the sense of letting go."
- "Music, I love it."
- "At the very end of the weekend, I look at my week ahead and make sure I schedule seeing friends or family, people who I like being with and who I value."

Try revisiting the daily appreciation exercise (Chapter 1, page 17). Over days, weeks, months, and years you can notice patterns in what you appreciate. Choosing to live with joy, ease, and meaning is to integrate these intentionally into your life.

LING: *It's people, at work, in my family, and friends. I have a small group of friends, no more than six people who I love and who love me. That's what's most important to me. There's another single mother—her kids are roughly the same age as mine, she's my best friend, we're in the same boat, we talk several times a week, and we get each other. Oh, and food—not cooking, eating.*

SAM: *For me it is my bike. I have several bikes now, one for riding to work and another for weekend rides. I'm rebuilding a classic steel road bike; oh and let's not forget the lightweight titanium road bike I drool over online even though my wallet is saying "no way you can afford that." There's something about the freedom a bike brings, you know? And working on my ride, that's a whole other level. It's like a therapy session with wrenches and gears.*

SOPHIA: *When I was working full-time, it was my work, my students, teaching, and my colleagues. I loved bringing as much light and laughter into my working day as possible. Now my dog is the best thing next to my children and grandchildren. Oh, and traveling to beautiful, interesting places when I can. With Parkinson's I appreciate my health, obviously. Actually, as I get older there is more and more I really appreciate.*

MOHAMMED: *For me sports, more following and watching now than doing. My wife, kids, and extended family of course. My faith.*

Your True North, Your Values

When you get to the end of each day and reflect on the day that's just passed, how often have you prioritized what is most important to us? On New Year's Eve, when you reflect on last year, how often have you prioritized what is most important to you for the year ahead?

> **PRACTICE:**   **Being with Your Future Self**
>
> *You can follow along on our website.*
>
> After taking a moment to gather and settle yourself, bring to mind your future self. This is you in the future, living with a sense of joy and ease. Keep it simple; sharpen the image of this version of yourself. Tune in to what happens as your future self comes alongside you, like a good friend. See if you can feel their presence, with a sense of care and protection. This good friend sees you and allows you to be exactly as you are, without conditions or judgment. When you're ready, see if they have anything they'd like to say to you about living well, with a sense of your true north, prioritizing what you value. Take your time, just see what comes up, and if nothing comes up, that's fine too.

MOHAMMED: *Growing up, I wanted to be a big-deal athlete, playing at the top level, including all the money and lifestyle I imagined that would bring. Many of my friends wanted to be celebrities—they all had someone they knew who had made a lot of money somehow by being a celebrity. We all wanted that lifestyle. But it's an illusion; if something seems too good to be true, it probably is. My true north is my faith, my family, and my sports team. That's it.*

Juggling the Balls in Your Life

There are times when living intentionally, with a sense of our true north, can seem like a luxury. Our lives are full, and we're surviving with little sense of the possibility of thriving.

EXERCISE: **Juggling Life**

You can follow along on our website.

Imagine that you are juggling all the major balls in your life. What are they? Work, your health, your finances, your friends, your values, your family, children? Which are most important to you? What would happen if you dropped one of these balls, short-term? Would it just bounce back unharmed? Would it be okay to sit out the juggling for a while? Would the dropped ball get a bit damaged but be reparable, or would it shatter irreparably? What about longer-term? Same questions, but now with a focus on the effect of dropping any balls over months or even years.

Living Well
by Finding Balance in Real Life, for Life

Finding balance was the focus of the last chapter. Living well is also about finding balance in what you prioritize, how you spend our time, and with whom. There are priorities we simply can't drop—financial security, childcare. There are those that, if we neglect them, could be damaged, perhaps a relationship. There are those that we'd miss but can pick up again later, perhaps interests or hobbies.

Balancing our lives is also an ongoing exploration. Sometimes you need to do less, sometimes you can do more, and sometimes you need to make changes in your life.

Taking Care of Our Relationships

The Barefoot Professor: Relationships

We're all part of a family, the *Homo sapiens* family. In the deepest sense of our biology and evolutionary story, we're social animals. That means we have evolved very high-level skills that help us function as part of a group. That is why being ostracized is so painful, loneliness so debilitating, and solitary confinement is one of the worst punishments in prisons. So, it should be no surprise that one of the largest long-term studies reveals that relationships are key to a happy life. Starting in 1938, it has tracked a large group of men over more than 80 years. Professor Robert Waldinger at Harvard Medical School, the current study lead, says it shows that good relationships are one of the most important determinants not only of happiness but also of health and longevity. Why? Other people provide us with connection, emotional and practical support, companionship, laughter, and so much more. And, of course, we provide this to others too. In short, a network of good relationships is key to well-being.

We need to take care of relationships just like we take care of everything else that we value. Whether it is family, friendship, or colleagues at work, our relationships require cultivation and sustenance. How do we take care of the relationships in our lives?

Mindfulness in Relationships

You can extend much of what you've learned about mindfulness to relationships. For example, attention can enrich your relationships. One of the most precious gifts you can give anyone is your full and undivided attention. If your attention is imbued with qualities of curiosity, kindness, care, acceptance, and patience, it can transform those relationships. More than this, these qualities can be cultivated through relationships. For example, intentionally bringing an attitude of appreciation and gratitude for the people in your life creates a sense of their value, which is the basis for respect, kindness, and generosity. To be seen, appreciated, and accepted is what helps children develop into adults who can manage their emotions and form securely attached relationships. It is what is needed for long-term romantic relationships, friendships, and professional relationships, not only to develop but also to evolve over time. It is what makes schools safe places for learning and workplaces sustainable places for productive work.

Sometimes, particularly over time, the focus in relationships can drift to what you don't like or what irritates us in others. Criticism, and in extreme forms coercive control and contempt, damages relationships and inevitably affects everyone's mental health. Similarly, in schools and workplaces, focusing exclusively on attainment and performance, without providing a climate of safety, respect, and trust, is not sustainable long-term. These negative climates alongside excessive demands are associated with poor mental health, absenteeism, fatigue, and burnout.

SOPHIA: *As a teacher, I saw my first task with any new class, especially at the start of the school year, was to create a positive culture. Where everyone felt safe, able to speak, and not speak if they chose not to, where there were boundaries and respect, me to them, them to me, and them to one another. Without this learning is not possible. Then I'd take time to get to know each young person and as far as possible make the class able to accommodate all their different ways of learning, strengths, and growing edges. I saw my job as offsetting and protecting them from some of the stuff they had to deal with elsewhere. I danced to my own tune, I admit it, but I had snacks for the kids I knew would not have had breakfast, I had a zero tolerance policy on any banter that made anyone feel unsafe, phones were in bags for the duration of the lesson, and I wove in lots of practices to help the class settle, focus, build a sense of playfulness, remind people to be kind, and so on. At the start of the year it was uphill, countercultural but often, especially as I trusted myself more over the years, by the end of the year the class would come in and know that was what to expect. I don't like to blow my own trumpet, but I could see for many of them it was like a sigh of relief when they entered my class.*

The Ancient Oak:
The Power of Attention and Presence in Relationships

In 2010 the artist Marina Abramovic put on an exhibition at the Museum of Modern Art in New York called *The Artist Is Present*. She sat across from an empty chair. Over the course of three months, eight hours a day, more than a thousand people sat opposite her. She lifted her eyes and met the gaze of each person, with steadiness and presence. By the end of the three months, there were lines of people snaking out of the museum waiting to take their turn. Some of the words they used to describe their experience were "moving," "luminous," and "profound." Many were moved to tears. Some said it was the first time in their lives they had encountered this quality of presence from another human being.

Much of what we've learned so far can help us relate to other people. If we listen carefully, our body and mind will tell us when we're safe, when our place in our "tribe" is secure, where we sit in hierarchical structures, who we are attracted to as friends or sexual partners, when someone needs us, when we need someone, what is needed in any given moment. Relationships go well beyond words to *how you are* with people. Coming home to your body (Chapter 3), the 50–50 practice (Chapter 3, page 65), and acts of kindness (Chapter 7, page 133) all support this work.

SAM: *My last partner ended our relationship just before our one-year anniversary—it stung like crazy. But you know, probably I should have listened to some red flags months earlier. It's like, over time, he started dialing back the presence—from 90%, then 80%, eventually hitting 50%. I could be right there with him and still feel lonely. I kept making excuses: "He's busy; he's got a lot on his mind."*

MOHAMMED: *We have traveled quite a lot with our kids, including some long plane journeys to visit my family. When the kids were really little, I remember when they started getting irritable after a while on an airplane, wanting to get out of the seat and crying. We'd talk to them and say things like "The man says we have to wear our seat belts," "If we can stay still until those lights go off, we can have a treat," "Here is another cartoon to watch," and so on. But none of this really worked for long. What worked when they were really little was holding them, rocking them, singing to them, helping them fall asleep. And if that didn't work, riding it out and being kind to ourselves by taking turns looking after them and realizing that this was difficult but time limited. A sense of humor too. We laughed so much on one trip when we found ourselves seated next to two children aged about seven or eight in economy class, whose parents had booked themselves into business class! By the end of the flight these two kids were helping us with our babies, and I had the sense they wanted to get off the plane with us, not their parents. So funny.*

Finally, in your relationships you can start to have a sense of the space between stimulus and reaction, where your values shape what you say and do.

MOHAMMED: *My wife and I have always talked. Before we got married, we spoke about both wanting kids, after my career-ending injury how she would be the primary breadwinner and I would stay home to raise the kids. We love each other, and I knew she wanted to have kids with me, and that included the me that was not an athlete.*

I have learned so much from her; she keeps these conversations alive in all the small moments in between. We were at the swimming pool when both kids were small, and I really wanted to swim—I mean work out and swim laps. She said she'd take the kids in the shallow kiddy pool while I did that. But the youngest was clingy and tetchy—he didn't want me to leave—and I heard this inner voice say "Mohammed, it's selfish to leave the kids." My instinct was to give in to that voice. When I offered to stay, she said, "Mohammed, you are a good dad, and I know what keeps you sane. Go swim. I can handle it." I couldn't see the space, but she could. We're a good team.

Again, you can revisit all of the ideas about reactivity and responding wisely (Chapters 6 and 9) with relationships in mind.

Healthy Relationships

When are relationships healthy, nourishing, fun, and rewarding? How do you take care to ensure you have the right relationships in your life?

EXERCISE: **What Relationships Nourish You?**

Bring to mind the main people in your life: friends, family members, neighbors, colleagues, or pets—those who are important to you. List them on a sheet of paper and then go through the list and ask, "Does each relationship nourish or deplete me?" If a relationship nourishes you, draw an arrow pointing up next to that relationship: ↑. If a relationship depletes you, draw an arrow pointing down next to it: ↓. A relationship may well have an element of both, being both nourishing and depleting. Feel free to draw as many ↑ and ↓ arrows next to them as seem to capture the balance of the relationship. Some may be neutral, neither nourishing nor depleting you; that's fine—just leave them as they are.

As you work through the list, ask yourself, "What is it that makes these relationships nourishing or depleting?" "What makes each relationship feel most healthy?" "What makes the relationship have a sense of mutual respect and trust?" With some of the key people in your life, think back to the last few times you have been together: "What was it like? What did you like and enjoy?" And over the last month, or earlier in the relationship, anything else? "What helps make this a healthy relationship?" Is it small acts of kindness, listening, doing things together that you both enjoy, laughter, honesty? To fill the list out further, maybe scan back over the last few weeks, months, even years. Ask yourself, "Is there anything else that makes these relationships stronger?"

This exercise builds on the earlier taking care of yourself inventory to include your relationships. It throws light on which relationships nourish you and perhaps also how they do this.

You can choose to commit to the relationships that nourish you and work to make them stronger. You can cultivate attention and attitudes of mindfulness in these relationships. The most rewarding relationships nourish us, but also explore deeper places, our foibles, vulnerabilities, and darker corners. Almost everything I have covered so far comes into play in these relationships, appreciation (Chapter 4), skillful response (Chapter 9), and equanimity (Chapter 10). Can you truly appreciate the people in your life, summon the courage to make changes, especially to how you are, accept what can't be changed, forgive, be open, guarded, boundaried—and have the wisdom to know what is needed in any moment? When someone else invites us into their lives, their world, it is a privilege, a place to practice these qualities of friendship. One of the most profound lessons here is the extent to which how we befriend those whom we love mirrors how we befriend ourselves.

> The litmus test of a healthy relationship is how we feel when we're with that person.

SOPHIA: *When I got my first senior leadership role in my school, I went on a weekend training course with other teachers making the same transition. It was called "inside out and outside in leadership," and we covered the idea of teaching authentically, with a realism about the many pressures on teachers, children, and leaders in schools. I was brilliant at being a good listener, skillfully drawing out the others in the course about their fears about this transition to being a leader. I'd gone into being a good carer role!*

Then I had a realization that made my stomach lurch. It was the first time that I glimpsed that what I thought was just me—a powerful inner critic—was something lots of teachers have. The weekend course included a lot on self-care, and there was something very powerful about a group of us, all teaching in bustling schools, starting the day with a healthy breakfast and some yoga, meditation, or a walk in the grounds. We laughed a lot, and the person facilitating the weekend course helped us connect with our inner critic in a new way, knowing it has good bits—our intention to be a good teacher—and letting go of the problematic bits, beating ourselves up about mistakes. We formed small peer groups over the weekend and stayed in touch after the course—I am still in touch with mine regularly, even though I'm retired now.

The Barefoot Professor:
What Makes for Healthy Relationships?

There is a lot of research and clinical experience about what makes for unhealthy relationships. The list is quite long: feeling unsafe, control and coercion, criticism and contempt, differing values, poor boundaries, poor communication, unresolved conflict, and lack of trust. Often these difficulties stem from previous relationships, especially unresolved difficulties and trauma. Much of what's been said about interest, presence, kindness, care, playfulness, values, trust, and responding wisely is important in good relationships. I'd maybe add good communication, having good times together, trust, respect, managing transitions and difficulties well, and asking for help if needed from others.

SOPHIA: *My partner and I are both a bit older, we've both had long relationships, and mostly figured out who we are, including what we value and like, as well as the inevitable baggage we've acquired along the way. For me being able to love him late in life involved realizing he was who he was, the good, the bad, all of it; he came with a richness of life, but also scars, a dad bod, and yes, some habits that I found grating— anything he washed up, he left on the draining board—he'd smile cheerily and say, "We can just grab glasses from the draining board." Raising my kids, my marriage, and teaching taught me an incredibly valuable lesson. Everyone is different, has their own needs, character, talents, growing edges, and weaknesses. Any relationship is about honoring all of it, allowing—no, enabling—people to be themselves. And asking that they do the same for you. I love his dad bod, even the cluttered draining board, because he smiles lovingly when he sees me eating peanut butter straight out of the jar. (Smiling) Just so as long as he understands I can only sleep on the side of the bed nearest the bathroom.*

EXERCISE: **How We Relate to Other People**

Imagine that today you are going to meet someone extraordinary, someone you admire, someone you would love to spend time with. They could be alive or dead. Perhaps someone like Nelson Mandela, Mother Teresa, Reese Witherspoon, Justin Timberlake, Malala Yousafzai, Jane Austen, Pele, Marie Curie, Muhammad Ali, or Greta Thunberg. Or if you are religious, someone from your religious tradition, a reincarnation of Mohammed, Rūmī, Jesus. But here is the thing: they won't reveal themselves. They could be someone at work, someone who works in your local shop, someone you say hello to as you both go about your day.

How would this change how you act around other people?

Now imagine everyone had the same idea. How would this change the world?

When We Are Caregivers: Compassion for Ourselves and Others

The Ancient Oak: The Story of the Two Acrobats

There is a Buddhist story where a master and student acrobat are training together. The master says to the student, "You take care of me, and I'll take care of you, and that way we'll both be safe." But the student disagrees and says, "No, that will not do. You look after yourself, and I will look after myself. That way we'll both be able to work together and stay safe. That's the right way to do it."

Throughout our lives we will find ourselves caring for others, as parents or looking after loved ones who need care because of a disability. As we and those we love live longer, we may need to look after elderly parents.

SOPHIA: *My husband and I raised our two kids; that was probably 22 years in total. Then my husband and I had a few good years before he became unwell. I cared for him for 8 years before he died. In the last 10 years of my mother's life, she needed more and more care, and because I lived closest, I did most of it. In the last few years of her life, her memory was devastated by her Alzheimer's disease. When I was exhausted and really struggling, my mother eventually moved into a residential care home with 24-hour nursing care, where she lived out the last 2 years of her life; I still visited her most days. Now I take care of Noah, my grandson, one day a week. When I look back, I'd say I have spent most of my adult life caring for someone.*

Caring asks a lot of us—attending to someone's distress, showing empathy, and responding to their needs. Care is part of the fabric of a relationship. It can also be depleting and, in extreme forms, lead to compassion fatigue. It is not a good idea or a luxury to take care of ourselves if we are caring for others. It is essential. We have to find a way of ensuring our own batteries are sufficiently charged not only to care for others but also to have enough perspective to know what care is needed and how it might best be provided.

> SOPHIA: *Having cared for people throughout my life, I've had to accept that I am going to need care myself. After I got the diagnosis of Parkinson's disease, I had a difficult decision. It was a recurring theme in my thoughts in my morning mindfulness practice over several weeks. I talked to someone I really trust about it. I still teach mindfulness programs. In a way, since receiving the diagnosis, my sense of service to and common humanity with my clients feels deeper; there were often others with chronic and progressive illnesses in the classes. When I introduce myself to clients, I briefly say something about my health status. The sense of common humanity and shared journey is strong in those moments—we are on this journey together. But as I became more aware of my need to take care of myself, I decided to recruit a co-teacher to help me teach the mindfulness courses. Then a year or two later, when I felt I was no longer well enough to teach, I moved to being a participant in the monthly mindfulness classes for all the people who have graduated my mindfulness classes. My co-teacher took over all my teaching. I had to let go of being a teacher and allow myself to be nourished by being a participant. I hadn't expected this, but my co-teacher became a friend, and I love seeing her develop what used to be my business into her own.*

Going through the Transitions in Life

Throughout our days and lives, we move through transitions, some of which we mark (birthdays, weddings) and others that we don't. Some are inevitable (births, changes in health, aging); some are welcome (meeting someone and falling in love), and some unwelcome (accidents, deaths, disasters, world events). Transitions can be important moments of awareness, appreciation, taking stock, celebration, acceptance, grieving, and learning.

Lengthening life expectancy means many of us have to navigate changes and transitions that our grandparents probably did not. Menopause, the transition to retirement, seeing children and grandchildren grow old, marriages ending, blended families, living longer into retirement, living longer with chronic illnesses, the deaths of family and friends—these are all transitions more and more of us will go through.

Many traditional stable societies mark transitions with rituals and ceremonies—the obvious ones of birth, marriage, and death, but the less obvious ones too, of puberty, for example. This ceremonial marking is important for many reasons. It makes the transition explicit, helps everyone have a shared understanding, and provides a chance to process the changes and make the necessary adaptations. But we have seen an erosion of some of these traditional societies and a whole set of new transitions. Perhaps we need some new ways to manage these transitions. In large and small ways, transitions are places to pause and ask what is important here, what is needed (see Chapter 9, page 185).

PRACTICE: **Moments of Transition**

One of the benefits of a regular mindfulness practice is to help you keep track of the state of your mind and body. This is both in any moment and in terms of themes across days, weeks, and months. Around transitions this helps you answer questions like "How am I with this?" "What is my body telling me?" "What emotions are around?" "Are there any calls to action?" "Are there any images or thoughts?" "What keeps coming up for me?"

SAM: *Coming home from work is like a whole playing field to navigate. The feelings from the day are swirling around, my neck and shoulders tight as a drum—all I want to do is zone out. Realizing how wound up I was and how much needed processing was part of the game. It hit me: I never asked myself, "How do I leave work at work?" I'd stroll in, wired and tired.*

I had to learn to make that shift from work to home. Walking out of the hospital, really leaving it behind, then hopping on my bike for the ride home. Stepping into my flat, telling myself, "This is home, time to kick back." The rest? Slowing down, maybe cooking up something healthy and actually enjoying the process, a hot bath, a call to a friend or the folks, or hitting the pavement for a run or bike ride. I won't front; it's hard, I often slip into zoning out, but even in those moments, I try to keep a thread of awareness. I mean, I'm not gonna game into the small hours on a work night. This was when I first downloaded a mindfulness app and then joined a face-to-face program for staff on learning to deal with stress. I was one of the youngest people there, but they were all tackling the same issues.

MOHAMMED: *My back injury changed everything. One day I was enjoying life as a college athlete on track to realize my dream of turning pro. Everyone on campus, or so it seemed to me, followed the team and would say "hi." After my injury I was in denial for months, maybe even years, trying everything, and getting multiple opinions from doctors, physiotherapists, sports scientists— anyone I thought might have the answer first to cure and then, when I realized that wasn't possible, for the pain. It was my dark night of the soul. I became my tormentor. "My body has let me down, I can't imagine a life without sports, I'm finished, I have no friends outside sports, my parents shared my dream, they are so disappointed in me." It was a plain-speaking specialist who told me that the breaks in my back meant I would never be able to be an athlete, and more than that I would have to learn to live with the pain. I sat in my car in the parking lot after the appointment and tried to gather myself. As I settled into my breath and body, I started to give myself a talking-to. "I have tried so many different things. I trust this doctor. That means I am going to have to face up to this. It feels really hard; it wears me down, makes me feel helpless and hopeless." Ironically, it was some of the stuff I'd learned as an athlete about putting down the negative self-talk and focusing on what was in front of me. "For now, I just have to deal with this moment, then drive home."*

A regular mindfulness practice can then also be helpful in several other ways: stabilizing, understanding, cultivating attitudes, setting intentions, and responding wisely.

MOHAMMED: *In my daily mindfulness practice I would sometimes get the thought, "I don't know who I am anymore. Who is Mohammed?" It was scary, but because it was coming up in a place that felt steady, it was okay, and I'd meet it with "It's okay; you've got this." I'd end my practice with the phrases "Open, curious, patient, and accepting," which helped me cultivate these attitudes and then set an intention for the day. "Today, take care to note what I enjoy, what is meaningful, when I felt good about myself." I realized that being a husband and father is really important to me. I was going to have to put myself back together as much for my wife and our kids as for myself. It has taken a few years, but I have a sense of who Mohammed is again.*

Some transitions have not been recognized, and others have been misunderstood or have even been seen negatively. In the last few years a generation of younger people has questioned traditional views of gender identity and demanded recognition of a wider set of possibilities beyond identifying simply as male or female. Women experiencing miscarriages during pregnancy have often borne this alone, but it is becoming easier to talk about and share with others. These are moments that need compassion and understanding. Menopause is becoming better understood, which in turn means it can be navigated better, by both the women going through it and everyone else.

SOPHIA: *I was overjoyed when I met my first grandchild at the maternity unit. On the drive home, though, I got a call from my son-in-law telling me that the baby was seriously ill and being moved into intensive care. Memories of losing my own child years earlier flooded back as if it were happening again right then. I felt nauseous; I was reeling with shock and worry. I turned my car around and headed back to the hospital. As I drove back through the shock and nausea, I prepared to launch myself into the project of my grandson's recovery.*

Over the next week, I spent many hours each day sitting with the baby. I started knitting—a cliché, I know [laughing]. I started by doing baby clothes for my grandson, but then I did them for other babies in the unit. Then I thought, "Oh, it's time to do something for me," so I did a hat and scarf. It's strange, I know, but I loved it, being there with him, absorbed in my knitting.

The unit started to become a place of sanctuary. It was so quiet—the babies were too ill to cry, and the nurses took care to speak in hushed voices, to close doors quietly, and to tend to the babies with extraordinary care. I found myself drawn into the stillness, the way the nursing staff seemed to embody love in action. They listened wholeheartedly to our worries, and in the midst of all the heartache around them the nurses moved with a calm dignity. That sort of gave me permission to sit for hours simply stroking the baby's hand and quietly singing and whispering to him. It was, I realized, the greatest gift I could offer to myself and my family: my daughter, my son in-law, and now my grandson, Noah. Even in the midst of this most challenging situation, I could be fully present with my grandson. I could even be fully present to all the uncertainty of his illness: What was it? Would he be okay? I was even able, in the midst of it all, to meet the memories of losing my own baby years before with compassion.

TROUBLESHOOTING: **Living Well**

I don't know what living well looks like for me. It helps to approach this in a spirit of curiosity and playfulness. As you go through your days, take time to tune in and ask, "What charges and what depletes my battery?" Broaden this out to ask about your values: "What adds value to my life? What is meaningful?" Rather than your life being a series of *have-to-do*s, it is possible to see what you enjoy, what adds value and is meaningful, not only for us, but the people you care about and the world you live in.

Exploring our relationships in terms of nourishment and depletion is not without risk. The lens of who we are will shape how we see our relationships, especially for someone brought up in a family without secure loving relations. It can also be quite evocative for someone with a history of trauma. But it can be important, because the quality of our relationships can determine the quality of our lives.

LING: *I used to be, still can be, mistrustful of everyone. In the early days of my marriage I would have sworn blind that my ex-husband was great, even though pretty much everyone had warned me about him. If I did this exercise when I was feeling tired and fed up, I'd probably write off everyone in my life. So I save it for when I'm in a good space, and I land on the question, "Are you sure?" when I just don't know if it's me or them that makes the friendship tricky with certain people. So I am trying to see if I can stay curious and open.*

Cultural values. Some cultures value busyness, self-sacrifice, denying pleasure, or subjugating needs. "You're busy! Good for you." "Don't be selfish." "That's self-indulgent." "You have to be a good daughter, wife. . . ." Again, a quality of curiosity and questioning can help us see when these cultural values serve us and when they don't, and how to work with them wisely.

Be open-minded. It is easy to get into ruts, where we do what we've always done. When we food-shop, we may always buy the same things; when we go on our phone, we have our favorite apps; when we watch TV, we have our favorite shows; with friends we have the same conversations; and so on. Maybe this serves us; maybe it doesn't. Try being open-minded: buy different food, try different shows on TV, ask friends questions you might not normally ask.

Don't expect miracles. Living well isn't some utopia. It may be your life doesn't change dramatically. It can be subtle, but if you pay attention, you will see the effects.

Patience. Creating the conditions for living demands patience. Cultivating new habits takes persistence and time. If you're exhausted or burned out, or breaking free from addiction, recovery takes time.

Living Well and Sustainably for Life

As I write this, I am in Kyoto looking out at a garden in autumn. Japanese gardens are famously places that create a sense of being at one with the natural world of plants, trees, streams, ponds, and mountains. They create a sense of ease, beauty, and contentment. That's because they were planned to have this effect and then cultivated with extraordinary care. Living well is what happens when you ensure the right conditions are in place for your mind, body, and life. But as with a Japanese garden, you have to continue to provide this cultivation throughout your life, adapting to the inevitable changes in your life.

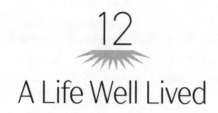

A Life Well Lived

Being the change you'd like to see in the world
—MAHATMA GANDHI

I started the book with these words and the promise that we would explore what they mean in your life. I hope that you have come to see that these are not just words; they point to a way of living aligned with your values. As you worked through the first 11 chapters of this book, you probably found that learning mindfulness for life, like anything else new, can seem unfamiliar and forced at first, but then becomes easier, although it still requires concentration and effort. In time and with practice, integrating mindfulness into your life becomes easier.

SOPHIA: *Through school and college I was driven, and if I'm honest I am not even sure what was driving me. I did well, trained as a teacher, did everything I was supposed to, more or less when I was supposed to, had friends, had a boyfriend, graduated high school and then college, got married, had a daughter. But if you asked me back then, "What does a life well lived mean to you?" I'd have scoffed at you— "No time for navel gazing; get on with it." Looking back on myself as a 22-year-old embarking on my career as a teacher, I can smile with a sense of "Bless, you were doing the best you could." So much of what I learned at school and in teacher ed has moved on so much. What was the point of all that calculus and mastering the overhead projector? But my mindfulness practice, which I've been doing just as long and it is now part of my life, as essential as eating, exercising, and sleeping, has never gotten old. It's taught me how to use my mind, to focus, be curious, present to myself and others, and joyful. It's still a work in progress, of course.*

Over months and years mindfulness can become second nature, even who you are and how you live. Inevitably, you will have setbacks and revert to old familiar habits. But that is part of learning how you'd like to be in the world, how you live your life. Staying on a mindful path through life, living according to your values to be the change you'd like to see in the world is what we'll turn to in this final chapter.

What Does It Mean to Be the Change You'd Like to See in the World?

This question invites you, over and over, to wake up (Chapter 1), pay attention (Chapter 2), come home to and really inhabit your body (Chapter 3), contemplate the preciousness of life (Chapter 4), and explore your aspirations and values (Chapters 1 through 11). You know deep in your being when your thoughts, words, and actions create contentment, meaning, and joy. And equally when they don't. That is what it takes to keep learning and evolving. You have started charting a route map, based in your values, and living in ways that line up with your deepest aspirations. This means how you respond to the people and world around you, but also how you are, what you say and do. It is very personal, but also deeply concerned with the people around you, your relationships, communities, and the wider world.

> *The Barefoot Professor and the Ancient Oak:*
> *Learning Complex Skills*
>
> **The Barefoot Professor:** There is a lot of research on how expertise develops. By way of example, I'll draw on the composer, conductor, and teacher Benjamin Zander again. Here he is describing what it looks like for people to become musicians. At first playing music is very labored and full of mistakes. Then it starts to come together but has a feeling of being played to a score, which of course it is. At this stage, mistakes can easily derail the player. When musicians become accomplished, the music sounds like it's being played through them—it has a life of its own and sounds natural, uplifting, and full of love. The psychological research on expertise and learning complex skills bears this out.
>
> **The Ancient Oak:** That makes a lot of sense. It reminds me of the teacher Ram Dass, who described learning as being like a tree growing. When it is a seedling, it needs protection from animals that might forage on it. When it grows into itself, it can stand strong and build connections with the woodland around it. In maturity, it may grow to provide shelter to other trees, plants, and animals.

Learning mindfulness for life doesn't follow a simple or straight line. Nor does it lead to some unrealistic perfect state. It includes embracing our reactivity—the inevitable mistakes, dark thoughts, mean impulses, the times we misspeak, and the oblivion of distraction. You start to have an awareness of these moments with qualities of interest, care, and openness to learning, even if they are difficult because you feel upset, guilty, lost, or ashamed.

> Practice is life, life is practice.

SAM: *When I first came out as gay, I was freaked out about how people might respond, and honestly, I worried about facing some attacks. It's a reality. So, what did I do? Signed up for Jiu-Jitsu classes. I'm all about it. No clue if I'd be able to use it for real, but my ninja vibe, the way I carry myself, the walk—maybe even a little swagger—it just makes me feel like I own it, you know? Like I'm less likely to be a target.*

MOHAMMED: *Sarah, my wife, knows that if I am upset about something, I get into a funk. She knows that it normally calms down. This afternoon, she took the kids to the zoo, leaving me to be grumpy by myself, knowing it would probably have blown over by the time they got home. It had, and later, when the kids were in bed and we were watching TV like two exhausted zombies, which we were, I reached out to hold her hand and said, "I'm sorry to be grumpy earlier." She smiled, kissed me, and said, "Let's talk about it when we're not both exhausted." (Smiling)*

Making Mindfulness Practice Part of Your Life

Mindfulness practice, like a lifelong friend, becomes an integral part of your life.

EXERCISE: How Does Mindfulness Practice Enrich Your Life?: Revisiting Your Values and Intentions

You can follow along on our website.

As ever, start with taking a moment to stabilize and steady yourself, with a sense of coming home to your body. When you are ready, remind yourself, "What is most important in my life? What or who do I value most?" With each idea that comes up, note it, then see what else comes up.

When you've made a list, ask, "How can my mindfulness practice help me?" "How can it support me with what I value most in my life?" Again, note each reason down, then ask the question again and see what else comes up.

This list is what transforms your practice from being something to build into your life to being something that helps you live the life you aspire to. Why do people practice mindfulness?

SAM: *I love being a ninja. Between my practice and throwing down in martial arts, it's like my inner ninja gets unleashed.*

LING: *To love unconditionally, starting with myself, then my kids, then my friends. To be brave, lean into what I love, not be pushed about by fear.*

MOHAMMED: *My family life is full-on, and every day can feel like a series of impossible demands, stresses, irritations, to-dos, ending with dropping into bed exhausted for a half sleep because the kids often wake us up. Frankly, with the nagging pain I live with, it is what makes it possible.*

SOPHIA: *I am living. I am dying. I want to do both well, and it helps me do that.*

Throughout we have outlined three forms of practice: mindfulness practice, everyday practices, and life itself. I'd like to revisit them with this idea of being the change we'd like to see in the world.

Mindfulness Practices for Life

I've introduced you to a whole range of mindfulness practices. Broadly speaking, you've used them for three different reasons. First, *to steady and stabilize yourself.* Traditionally, these are called *concentration practices,* and you'll have developed a sense of which practices work for you in different circumstances. Second, *to befriend your minds by cultivating attitudes of mind.* You're cultivating curiosity, appreciation (Chapter 4, pages 82–83), kindness, care, trust, effort, patience, letting go, courage (Chapter 7), and balance (Chapter 10). Third, *to develop understanding and wisdom.* As you will have seen, this emerges from your practice as you start to see the workings of your mind and body: the links in the chain of reactivity and steps needed to respond wisely (Chapter 9).

These different practices are like three legs of a stool; you need all three to give you stability and strength. You need some degree of focus to see what is happening and develop understanding. The attitudes of mindfulness broaden and build focus and understanding, but also emerge out of understanding. So, my invitation to you is to ask yourself what mindfulness practice is right for you today, this week, this month, this year. To trust that you know what you need. This includes knowing what is realistic, balanced with what you need. There may be periods where you choose to do a particular practice, periods when you practice intensively and consistently, and other times when you step back from mindfulness practice altogether.

SOPHIA: *I've had a mindfulness practice now for at least thirty years, and it is part of my life, as essential as eating, exercising, and sleeping. It has gone through many transitions. There was a time I felt out of contact with my body, and for months I did a particular form of yoga, and slowly but surely had a real sense of befriending my body but also strengthening it. When my kids were young, and there were a few years I was teaching full-time, I did much less mindfulness practice, but it felt like I had laid foundations and kept what I had learned going in other ways. After my husband died, I was scared to practice, scared that I'd be overwhelmed by loneliness and longing. So, I listened for and encouraged the small voice that suggested I needed to be patient, kind, brave, and look after myself. This shifted something for me; the loneliness was filled by thankfulness for who he was and what he'd been in my life. Over months and years, I started to be ready to start living again. It wasn't easy. The first time I made love with someone who wasn't my husband all I could do was think of him; it was awful. But with time I felt ready to love again. And with my Parkinson's, my mindfulness practice has been a life saver. It's given me the balance and courage to live while also preparing myself for the inevitable deterioration in my health. I have faith—it's the only word that seems right—that it will help me too with dying and all that will involve.*

Everyday Practices for Real Life

You've started to use a whole range of practices intended to bridge what can be learned from mindfulness practices into everyday life. In a sense this is simply about mindfulness practices being adapted so they can be used throughout your day. This applies to all the everyday practices I've introduced—the Breathing Space, appreciation, 50–50, but especially the practices that you have found most helpful. This may change over time, and having this sense of curiosity and openness means that you can learn and use different practices at different times.

Life as Practice

How the mindfulness practices support you in your life is what it's all about. There are so many ways you already bring awareness and attitudes of mindfulness into your day. Here are just a few:

  • From the moment you're born to the moment of your death, your body is with you. You've been becoming more aware of how your body moves through your day, your posture, your movement. This helps you remember to ask, "What does my body need in this moment?" How is your body when you move from lying down to sitting, to standing, to walking? Does it need anything, a shift in posture, a stretch, a shake-out, some exercise?

• Coming to your senses. The expression "coming to our senses" is so interesting. Your senses are your friend, your teacher, the bridge between your inner and outer world. Carry on being playful with your senses. For example, with hearing, see if you open to really hearing the notifications on your phone, a bird, traffic noise, the sound of a heater or air conditioner, laughter, the wind, muffled voices in another room. You can use any sound as a reminder to "come to your senses." Throughout your day, explore which senses are most in play; would it be interesting to intentionally engage other senses? Really listen, or taste, or see, or touch, or smell.

• You can always anchor yourself. You'll have developed a sense of what anchors work for you in different situations. Throughout the day, take a few moments to anchor yourself and how this affects your day.

• Eating and drinking are places to practice many aspects of mindfulness. At least sometimes, see if you can eat or drink and really savor the smell, taste, and texture. Besides savoring, you can also be curious and appreciate the many people and conditions that were involved in the chain of bringing the food and drink to you—the sunlight, the rain, the earth, the farmer, the trucker, the shop workers.

• Savor and appreciate good moments. Eating and drinking are low-hanging fruit to practice mindfulness. But you can savor, be curious, and appreciate all the pleasures in life, whatever they are for you—music, games, nature, sports, film, being with people, making love, being alone, reading, writing . . . .

• Our days have many moments we might see as "dead space." Standing in a line, commuting to school or work, waiting for the kettle to boil, anticipating before a meeting starts—these are all moments when it is possible to check in, anchor, and open your awareness. Can you notice what is happening with your breathing and body? Feel the contact points of your body with the world, your feet on the floor, your clothing. Anchor and with whatever attitudes seem right, open your awareness up.

• Befriend difficulties such as busyness, stress, and pain. In these moments, be aware of any points of tightness in your body throughout the day. Is there tension anywhere in your body? Your neck, shoulders, stomach, jaw, or lower back? See if you can breathe into them and, as you exhale, let go of excess tension. If possible, stretch or do some yoga once a day. Yes, a life without busyness, stress, and pain might seem idyllic, but given they are here, see if you can befriend them.

• Finally, if you ever feel jangled, overwhelmed, or like you have "lost it," remember that there is no failure, falling short, disappointing someone, or getting it wrong in being the change we'd like to see in this world. In any moment, you are starting over again, right here, right now. Any moment is a moment you can ask, "What does this moment need?" The analogy with friendship works again. For all sorts of reasons friendships ebb and flow, we're busy with work, family, or need time alone, but a good friend is there, and you can come back to them, and if necessary, talk honestly and openly about problems. Over time this builds trust and strengthens our friendships.

Exploring Ways to Practice and Learn with Other People

Finally, as we're social animals, practicing regularly with others is one of the most powerful ways to keep your practice vital. This is both for the obvious reasons that we can support and learn from each other, but also the less obvious reason that mindfulness practice with others opens a more collective awareness and understanding. Mindfulness practice alone has a different quality from mindfulness practice with others. Both can be valuable in different ways and at different times in our lives.

> MOHAMMED: *I wanted to keep my practice up, and going along to mindfulness classes occasionally reminds me how powerful the practices can be. I also like to chat to people a bit about what they're doing and get some new ideas. It kickstarts me and reinforces stuff in my brain.*

If you would like to learn mindfulness with a group, look out for opportunities for reunions and practice days (see the Mindfulness for Life website to find a group).

TROUBLESHOOTING: Questions and Obstacles in Integrating Mindfulness into Your Life, *for* Life

Integrating all these ideas and practices into our lives will inevitably throw up questions and obstacles. Each chapter has named and suggested some of the ways to work with the most common obstacles.

As we've discovered in each troubleshooting section, difficulties are not only to be expected. If we look carefully, they will teach us something.

First, we learn that mindfulness is not something we do—not another task, chore, or health measure per se but rather a resource that we all have and can use throughout life when we stop trying to "do it."

> LING: *I start and end every day with a to-do list. You know, the usual adult stuff like getting my car fixed. But I've learned to throw in things I actually enjoy, like hanging*

out with friends or treating myself to something special. When the day winds down, I look at the list. If I haven't checked off everything, I figure out when I can get to it. And if that nagging feeling of "You didn't ace today's to-do list" creeps in, well, there's the tough judge. Wasn't my plan, but it surprisingly helps me sleep better. Writing it all down means they don't ambush me in the middle of the night.

If you've let your mindfulness practice lapse, it could also be because you feel like the people around you don't get it and aren't supportive. Of course, sometimes the people around us or our circumstances can affect our mindfulness practice. Remind yourself that your practice is there to resource and nourish you. It is there to help you be in and navigate your life.

There is no guru or magical formula, nor can you will happiness into being. You could even say that chasing happiness often backfires because it creates a gap between how things are and how we think they should be, which creates striving and dissatisfaction. Gurus want us to think they have the answers that we need. Instead, what I am suggesting is first that you only trust what you experience directly for yourself as helpful. And that happiness, joy, contentment, wisdom, and the capacity to respond wisely are what emerges naturally in the course of a life lived well. You'll have to see for yourself if this is true for you.

MOHAMMED: *There is a cliché in sports that is a cliché for good reason. I remember my coach saying to me "In training, just focus on that training session and training for the next game. In the next game, just focus on that game. In that game, just focus on each moment. If you do that, everything—your selection for the team, your contract for next season, your career—will unfold by itself just as it is supposed to." I found this so helpful as an athlete, but in my life too.*

The Ancient Oak and the Barefoot Professor: The Story of the Child and Two Wolves

The Ancient Oak: There is a story of a child talking to a grandparent. "Sometimes I get really confused and stuck. I feel like I have these two different voices in my head, like two very different wolves. One of them is kind, loyal, and has my back; I trust it. The other is judgmental, impulsive, but can also be mean-spirted; also, it's exciting. I don't know which one is going to win out." The grandparent responds: "The one you feed, the one you pay most attention to, the one you give most time and energy to—that's the one that will become stronger, clearer, and louder." The child responds with a question that surprises the grandparent, "Yes I see. But can they be friends?"

The Barefoot Professor: As they say, "out of the mouths of babes." Combining different parts of our history and ourselves into a stable, authentic, and integrated self is one of the tasks of adolescence and early adulthood and goes on throughout our lives.

The Ancient Oak and the Barefoot Professor: Seeing, understanding, and befriending our minds is what helps these voices be seen for what they are and to become friends.

Being the Change
We'd Like to See in the World

All that we are now is a result of all that we have been; all that
we will be tomorrow will be the result of all that we are now.
—CHRISTINA FELDMAN AND WILLEM KUYKEN

Living According to Our Values
through How We Are and What We Say and Do

Understanding and cultivating our minds and bodies is a lifelong project. Everything we've covered can be explored with greater depth, again and again, and extended into new areas of life.

Everything Rests on the Tip of Intention

Intention comes out of our values, the compass that points us toward our true north.

The Ancient Oak: Intention and Values

In philosophy ethics are concerned with right and wrong, especially when our values are challenged. Contemplative traditions have language that is perhaps more helpful than *right and wrong*. In moments of choosing to respond, I prefer the words *helpful* or *healthy*, or *well-being*. That is to say, "What words or actions will be helpful here, for me, for others and the world? What will reduce suffering and enhance well-being?" And, of course, the flip side, unhelpful, "Are these words or actions unhelpful? Do they create suffering?"

> **PRACTICE:** **Revisiting Your Values and Intentions in an Ongoing Way**
>
> *You can follow along on our website.*
>
> Once you've gathered and settled yourself, bring to mind a majestic tree and have a sense of yourself as that tree. You are firmly rooted, in your values. Your roots spread out into the ground and draw on the soil. Remind yourself what brings you a sense of meaning and enduring contentment. Who or what is it in the world that gives you that sense of purpose and joy? What really matters? Stay with these questions, maybe asking them a few times to see if something more comes up as you ask them the second, third, fourth times.
>
> Your torso, like a tree trunk, legs, arms, neck, and head, like the branches and foliage, together they represent your understanding, your wisdom.
>
> Like water, infused with nutrients, your values pass up the tree as intentions, merging with your understanding and translating into words and actions.
>
> Out of this embodied understanding flows what you do and say. Like the tree, you can respond to the winds of changing conditions, while keeping your integrity.
>
> Imagine yourself as this majestic tree, in all sorts of conditions, able to adapt but nonetheless strong.
>
> This practice reveals our deeper values.

MOHAMMED: *My roots are my faith; that's what helps me be a good father, husband, son, and brother. (Smiling) And accept that my sports team hasn't won a tournament for years.*

What matters most is different for different people—perhaps family, work, connection with the natural world, financial security. But it can also reveal values that are shared in a family or community—respect for elders, being a good sport, individual rights, collective harmony. Finally, it can reveal values that are more universal, that few people would disagree with: help the people you love, return favors, divide resources fairly, and respect others' property. This idea of your personal, community, and more universal values provides your compass and is something that can be explored for a lifetime as you encounter new people and new situations and as you learn, through trial and error, what is most important.

Befriending Ourselves

We start with befriending ourselves, with a sense of coming home to our body, and not only knowing but also befriending our mind.

SOPHIA: *I was walking Rufus on the beach. There was this woman, about my age, doing the same, throwing sticks into the surf for her dog to retrieve. My dog wanted* to play and was chasing the stick too. The woman seemed not to care that Rufus had invaded her game. Then to my horror Rufus crouched down at the water's edge and emptied his bowels. I was horrified, not just because it was right by this woman and there were swimmers and surfers, but also because I had forgotten the bags to clear up his mess. Without pause, she used one of her bags and picked up my dog's mess. I went up to her expecting her to be rightly angry with me, and I was ready to apologize unreservedly. She waved away my apology, smiled, passed me the bag, and said, "Don't worry about it; we can't control when our dogs decide to empty their bowels." It was an extraordinary turning point for me, to see someone I could identify with so accepting, so kind, so nonjudgmental.

LING: When I am stuck in depression, it is like a swamp, darkness and a sense of rotting. My closest friends know to ask, "Ling, are you in your swamp?" We went on a family trip recently and visited a rain forest. It was beautiful. But what struck me most was that the swamp is incredible. It gives life to all the tropical flowers, insects, and animals that live there. Also, the swamp is an essential part of a larger rain forest that turns our CO_2 emissions back into oxygen. I try to remind myself that the swamp is just a small part of who I am, and I can step back and see the whole beautiful forest.

> The work of a lifetime is to befriend our minds and bodies, to see it, with all its many parts that make up an extraordinary whole.

Our Relationship with Ourselves as a Foundation for Healthy Relationships with Others

LING: One morning I went downstairs, and my teenage daughter was eating her breakfast, watching a show on her laptop computer, while also texting a boy. It was 10 minutes until she would need to head out the door to catch the bus to school, she'd left the bathroom light on, and there was a wet towel on the floor, the fridge was ajar, a container of milk was out on the counter, and a cereal box was open. I felt a wave of irritation and an impulse to say, "You have 10 minutes to eat your breakfast and then I need you to clean up after yourself in the bathroom and kitchen." When I was her age, I was living in foster care. This tripped my irritation into anger and the impulse to nag into an impulse to lash out: "What the hell do you think you're doing? I am not your slave; you're not leaving this trail of destruction for me to clean up when you go to school!"

I don't really know how, but I knew in that moment in my gut that if I said the words on the tip of my tongue, my daughter would roll her eyes, say something rude under her breath, make a half-hearted attempt to put a few things away, and then head out the door without a good-bye, leaving a dark cloud of resentment behind her. I felt helpless, and my mind started to go down a spiral of negative thinking: "I am *a terrible parent. When she leaves, I am gonna get back into bed." I bit my tongue, knowing that this was not a fight worth picking. As my daughter headed out the door I said, "Have a good day, I love you," and she looked back and smiled, saying, "Thanks, you too." She was oblivious to the drama playing out in my mind or the mess she was leaving behind.*

But when the door closed, I felt relief that I hadn't lashed out.

That evening, after school, I gave my daughter a ride to a friend's house. In the car, she opened up about what was on her mind, and I gave her lots of space and just listened. Driving home, I felt pleased and proud of my daughter. She is so much more together than I was at her age.

When you are awake to yourself, you cannot help being awake to others. If you are aware of your bodily sensations and thoughts, then other people's words, actions, and presence will also inevitably resonate in your awareness. As you've seen, in these moments you can choose to change perspective before responding (Chapters 8 and 9).

Kindness, compassion, perspective, and wise responding are needed more than ever. The problems in the world are complex and need us to work together. The migration of people around the world requires us to understand and communicate with people from different cultural backgrounds. It is possible to hold a sense of difference without creating outgroups, especially outgroups we judge to be more or less than us. Yet there are groups with vested financial, political, or ideological reasons for creating ingroups and outgroups, denigrating others, exploiting conflict, and other nefarious motivations.

Being able to see and respond with intentions, words, and actions that are healthy is much needed in the world. This happens in moments small and large throughout our day.

SOPHIA: *I was a good teacher. One of the most important things I did in my career was creating classrooms that were safe and fun. I don't want to be immodest, but I was good at it. Not only was this essential for the kids to learn, but for many I know my classroom was a sanctuary. For some school wasn't fun, for others home wasn't safe. I hope in some small way I gave these kids a sanctuary. Some of my former students keep in touch. One runs a boxing gym, and I know he runs it the same way—a lot of the kids in our community go there because it's home.*

I noticed toward the end of my career that schools became more and more pressured as assessments and exams became the be all and end all. One of the effects for us as teachers is that this pressure played out in every part of school life. It made creating a sanctuary in my classroom all the more important, and my peer group of senior teacher friends was also my sanctuary. That's part of why I didn't burn out or leave like so many of my colleagues.

MOHAMMED: *I was driving over the main bridge over the river when I saw this young man; something wasn't right. When I looked again, I saw he was on the outside of the guardrail facing the river. I pulled over and walked over, taking care not to get too close. He was a young man, Muslim, South Asian, dressed in a tracksuit, expensive trainers. Another older, white guy came up too and was on the other side of him. We both started to talk to him; it seemed natural knowing what to say, sensing not to pressure him. But I could see he could jump any moment. Somehow the other guy and I were on the same page. At a certain moment we both nodded and quickly grabbed him and dragged him over the guardrail to safety. He started to wail, like an animal, and the two of us just stood there holding him and talking to him. I could feel he had nothing on him, no bag or phone—he'd been serious about jumping. By now some other cars had stopped and someone had called the emergency services, which came not long after. They took over and took him to the psychiatric emergency room. The other guy and I stopped and talked for a while, and as we said goodbye, we embraced even though we'd never met before. Twenty minutes in my life where it felt like everything I'd come to understand from my Muslim faith, my mindfulness practice, my own life flowed naturally.*

LING: *I used to feel broken and damaged because of my upbringing. Who abandons their children like my parents did? What did that say about me? For years I assumed there was something wrong with me—that they had abandoned me because I was broken or defective in some way. But when I became a mother, I realized that wasn't possible. When I looked at my two children in my arms for the first time, all I saw were these unformed, vulnerable beings that needed more than anything to be loved. Yes, I was scared, but in that moment I decided that the most radical thing I could do was to do what wasn't done for me: show up for my kids as a mother, love them unconditionally, and never again be ashamed of who or what I am.*

Phases of Life and Transitions Again

To live is to change, and to live well is to change often.
—JOHN HENRY NEWMAN

The inevitable transitions you navigate throughout your life provide a chance to take stock, appreciate all that is well, and reset. Yet often these transitions are represented negatively. What is the first thought that comes to mind when you think about puberty, becoming sexually active, doing a midlife review, children leaving home, menopause, or moving into assisted living? *Midlife review* may well translate into "midlife crisis," menopause can be reduced to hot flashes, children leaving home is sometimes described as the "empty nest." But what happens if you really pause, with an open-hearted sense of interest as you move through these transitions? Every transition becomes a chance to "walk down a different street" or at least walk down a street avoiding the potholes.

SAM: *Back in the day they called me "skinny Sam." Seeing all the sporty boys and jocks in my school made me feel kinda inadequate. Well, you can imagine when I first started being attracted to men, I was worried that no one would find me attractive. Then I got together with this guy, one of my first partners; he was more experienced than me. I adored the guy, and he made me feel safe as I explored my sexuality. When we had sex, he loved my body and would tell me so. He dropped this bomb that my body shape was a particular tribe in the gay community. I wasn't skinny Sam wearing baggy clothes, boom—I was a "twink." Seeing my body through his eyes, seeing he wanted me as I am, did wonders for how I feel about my body. Years of wishing I looked more like the sporty popular guys at school went out the window. I switched up my wardrobe and started to strut my stuff a bit more. And you know what? Turns out it wasn't just him who found me attractive; that was a good feeling.*

Growing old can be seen as losing vitality and strength. Often, we rail against it with denial, gym memberships, and Botox. But we forget that just a few hundred years ago growing old was not something most people around the world experienced—in 1900 life expectancy across the world was less than 50. Aging is a privilege our forebears a few generations ago did not have. The attitudes we've cultivated—interest, kindness, care, courage, trust, equanimity—can help us see aging not only as a privilege but also as something to accept on its own terms, being open to what we see and learning when we do this.

LING: *My kids are growing up. They still need me, but not in the same way. I'm in a good enough place to start asking myself, as I start to have more time, what I want to fill it with. I'm not forcing it; I am leaning into it. When I stand in front of the mirror in the morning getting ready for the day, I see me, holding myself, all of it with appreciation, forgiveness, and, yes, love. I am mostly comfortable in my own skin, getting ready for a day that involves a job I am good at and my two kids, who I love. Yes, of course, I also see the lines on my face, some gray in my hair, the extra weight on my body, my belly that carried my two children to term. I found myself the other day saying to myself as I looked in the mirror, "Bless, she is gorgeous, strong and decent."*

Dying is a transition that understandably we avoid thinking about. It evokes fear, of pain, disability, of being unable to cope, to say nothing of the existential fear of death itself. We've explored how to open to and be with difficulty, and turning toward dying and death is a natural extension of these ideas. The same principles come into play of trusting the mind to know what is and what isn't possible, of anchoring, of moving toward and away from difficulty, of trusting the body as a home to come back to, as somewhere that can hold and process difficult experiences. And in a sense, we're always about to die. Each time we do something—read, text, walk, dance, make love—could be the last, which is why the moments, and inhabiting them, count. That's why awareness of death and dying can be helpful to living fully and well.

The Ancient Oak and the Barefoot Professor:
Contemplating Death

The Ancient Oak: There is a contemplation in Buddhism that involves thinking about our own death. This is not intended to be gloomy and depressing. Instead, it is intended to help us remember that it is our nature to age, get sick, and eventually die. The realization that good health is fragile and our time on earth is finite can help us appreciate our lives and commit to living life.

The Barefoot Professor: Many people who have faced their mortality because of an encounter with someone else who is dying, a life-threatening accident, or illness describe this experience of waking up to the preciousness of life. We can wake up in less dramatic ways than meditating on death. For example, there is some emerging research suggesting that cold-water swimming acts like a cold shock that wakes us up. The appreciation practice has much the same effect of helping us wake up to what is meaningful, good, and joyful in our lives.

Yes, some people die suddenly or in their sleep. We can be lucky to have palliative care and incredible drugs that can ease pain and make dying more comfortable, or even assist the dying process. But if we are lucky enough to live into old age, we will, more than likely, have to meet aging and death on their own terms: losing abilities and the body's functions slowing down, deteriorating, and eventually shutting down, often in ways that are distressing and painful.

SOPHIA'S DAUGHTER: *My mother died as she lived. She started every day with mindfulness practice if she was able, and I remember her telling me she was using phrases, sort of like prayers in her practice. "May I be safe and protected, open and courageous, and may I live with care for my own suffering and also those around me who care for me and who I love."*

Her world became smaller and smaller physically, first her home, then a few rooms of her home, then we had to move her to a nursing home, where she had just a room and a bathroom, and toward the end she didn't leave her bed. But I could see she kept what was important alive in her memory and in imagination. Of course, these moments became fewer, and she slept a lot. But when she was awake and with it, she let me, my brother, and her friends know, with a squeeze of the hand, a look, and words, that she loved us, she was okay, that she was rooting for us, that she wanted us to live our lives wholeheartedly after she was gone and that she felt she'd lived a good life and was ready to die. She died with me, my brother, her partner, a few of her friends, and Rufus in the room, as peacefully and well as any death can be. After she died, one of the nurses told me she'd said that she wanted her care plan to ensure not just that she was comfortable, but that those of us in the room also wouldn't find the inevitable changes in her declining vital signs and moment of death traumatic. Like I said, she died as she lived.

My son, Noah, adored his grandmother, my mother. They spent a lot of time together, and I learned later they'd read many books together, including about dying. Once he came home from school and announced, "We're all going to die like Nana, probably you first, then Dad, then Rufus, then me, but only in like a thousand years." I just smiled and said, "That sounds about right; we'd better make the best of it." He replied, "Yes, that's what she said. Can I have an ice cream? Me and Nana always had an ice cream."

My mother asked Noah to look after Rufus. It's worked so well. Rufus is so protective of Noah. He's a German shepherd, and the first thing Noah does when he comes home from school is hang out with Rufus. The other day he said, apropos of nothing, "Rufus is my best friend."

I can see much of my mother in Noah, even though he is still just a boy. She asked in her letter of wishes to have a memorial headstone with the phrase "A life well lived." Noah is doing that already, living his life well, I mean.

Taking Care of Our World

Just as Sophia was shaped by and shaped her world, so too are you. As you resource yourself and your relationships, you can extend your care through "widening circles of concern," the communities, organizations, and wider world, both now and in the future.

The Ancient Oak and the Barefoot Professor: Being Part of Something Larger

Melanie Challenger, scientist, writer, and broadcaster, argues in her book *How to Be Animal* that as human beings we're not that special or different; we are much more like other animals than we like to admit. Her argument can be expanded to wider ecosystems, the natural living world of other species, plants, forests, ocean life, and the health of our physical planet. And it can be expanded to time: planet earth is approximately 4.5 billion years old. Our species, *Homo sapiens*, has been part of that history for a fraction of that time,

200,000–300,000 years. Zooming out can help with changing our perspective. This is true given that we have accrued so much power that for the first time in our planet's history we are responsible for some of the seismic changes, for example, in biodiversity and climate.

The evidence for climate change is overwhelming. It is already affecting the world and could affect the next generation in profound ways. Inequalities across the world, in wealth, access to education and health care, for people of different sexes, genders, cultural backgrounds, and religions, cause tremendous suffering. Extraordinary technological innovation has brought many benefits, such as access to information, but also many challenges, the way information is misused and the reality that these technologies can create connection and alienation. These are challenges that must be addressed with urgency, with imagination, and through collective responsibility.

Albert Einstein put it like this: "Only the individual can think, and thereby create new values for society—nay, even set up new moral standards to which the life of the community conforms. Without creative, independently thinking and judging personalities, the upward development of society is as unthinkable as the development of the individual personality without the nourishing soil of the community" ("Why Socialism," *Monthly Review*). Or as Professor Jon Kabat-Zinn points out, regardless of how these problems came about, they will need to be solved by human minds and hearts. We can be optimistic because we know how to train the mind and heart.

How are you shaped by, and how can you shape, the world? How can we respond, individually and collectively, to the major challenges in the contemporary world? Again, this is a question where mindfulness practice, including in our everyday life, can help. Awareness imbued with interest will inevitably yield answers. More than this, it can make us feel uncomfortable in ways that are helpful. Guilt, frustration, and impatience can be teachers; they can tell us when we perhaps need to question our words and actions and do more, better. Anger can tell us about violations of boundaries, of trust, of power. Your values are your compass, and your mindfulness practice can provide the focus and energy needed to move forward. Responding skillfully applies beyond our immediate concerns to the wider world (Chapter 9, page 166) when we expand our questioning to "What will serve the well-being of the wider world?"

The Ancient Oak: The Story of Starfish Stranded on a Beach

In her book *The Star Thrower*, Loren Eiseley tells a story of a little girl and an old man walking on the beach after a storm when they come across hundreds of starfish washed up on the sand. The little girl picks one up and throws it into the sea. The man says, "There are so many; there is no way you can rescue them all." She replies, "That's true, but I saved that one." He joins her, and together they do what they can to save some of the starfish.

The scale of problems, negativity, and pessimism can seem overwhelming. We can feel small and ask, "What difference can I make?" But any change comes about only through words and action, and we have direct control only over our own words and actions. It was not so long ago that life expectancy was less than 50, that women around the world were not able to vote, that access to education and health care was for the privileged few. These seismic changes came about through the collective endeavor of many individual people like us.

LING: *After my divorce I got a job as a court reporter because the hours worked well with the school day. The work involved listening, every day, to criminal cases of sexual assault, rape, domestic violence, child abuse, and so on. I used to think that our gallows humor at work and not taking work home protected me from hearing all this stuff day in and day out. But I realized that it was just not a good place for me to work because it was bringing up a lot of memories and feelings—I was living in a state of constant high stress—I was outside the window of what I could manage.*

It took time, but I took a course in horticulture, worked as a volunteer at the botanical garden, and I loved it. Now I work in a local garden center run by a family who are passionate about gardening. I love learning about plants, flowers, and trees, taking care of them, and helping the customers. I'd like one day to run programs with young people in our garden center, the sort of young people who lose their way, who I used to see in the courts, and who I was too.

SAM: *It grinds my gears when old people say, "The future belongs to young people." Like, hold up, you created this mess, and now you're passing the burning torch to us? I'm all about the environment, and honestly, I am terrified that some really bad things will happen. That's why I bike everywhere and ditched eating red meat. I'm all about people's health and well-being, which is why I chose nursing. But let's be real, everyone's got a role to play, especially the ones who set it all on fire and have the power to do something about it.*

MOHAMMED: *I am taking courses in coaching. I want to coach youth athletics in our Muslim community, not because I hope to produce elite athletes. But because it's a place where young people can come together and learn so much that prepares them for their lives, about self-respect, discipline, teamwork, and so much more.*

SOPHIA (in her last journal entry): *The last few months of my life have brought me face to face with the questions of what I am proud of in my life, what I regret, and what was on my bucket list. I feel good about my work as a teacher, raising my kids, my marriage, caring for my husband and, even though it nearly broke me, caring for my mum. I don't regret anything. In the end I realized that there is only one thing that matters, to love and be loved. And I love seeing my former students, friends, and family passing it on.*

Mindfulness shines light on your mind and life, and this enables you to see and understand how you shape and are shaped by the world, in small and large ways. It provides a sense of steadiness. You can use what you've learned to develop perspective and tools for answering the question "What is needed?" It creates the sense of "We need to do something" that can energize and motivate us. It also creates a sense of common humanity. We are all part of the wider world, affected by it and able to shape it. With our values and all the skills we've learned, we have a chance to shape the world. Finally, mindfulness builds what psychologists call "intrinsic motivation," which translates as not only "I've got this" but also "I'm on it." And the courage to act.

Mindfulness in Real Life, for Life

Our lives are shaped by others—the people who raise us, the people who educate us, the people we work for, the people who want us to buy their products, and the people who need our support. If we live reactively, without awareness, we risk living someone else's idea of our life, which may or may not be in our best interests. As our awareness develops, this inevitably means coming to realize very directly all these ways that the world impacts us. Whether we are aware of it or not, the world's most pressing issues affect us directly and indirectly—climate change, an explosion of information, new technology that is driving many societal trends, the prevailing culture. This resonance may be urgent and loud, like someone living in an area where crops are failing because of water shortages, or persistent and pervasive, such as the algorithms feeding us information via our digital devices, or subtle but constant, as in the background pollution of a busy city.

Many of the pressing issues in our world will need to be solved by human minds and hearts. This is true for smaller, local issues in our lives, and the larger issues facing not only our generation but also future generations. There are reasons to be hopeful. Throughout history well-trained minds working individually and together have addressed major health problems like smallpox, HIV-AIDS, and most recently Covid-19. Our forebears learned to farm so people could rely on food being available year round. More and more people around the world are living in economic conditions that create financial and material security. Nations and international bodies have created treaties and structures for preventing wars and maintaining security.

Being the change you'd like to see in the world means keeping yourself, other people, and our planet in mind. It means using your values as a compass. It requires a route map from where you are to where you'd like to be. It requires curiosity, open-heartedness, and courage. It demands that you keep learning as you move through your life, and adapt as you move through life's inevitable transitions. Imagine an education that helps us develop the wisdom to see how things are, the imagination to see how we'd like them to be, and the creativity and courage to create the world we'd like to live in. The coming together of ancient wisdom and modern psychology that we've covered so far provides this education.

The Barefoot Professor and the Ancient Oak:
Endings and Beginnings

The Ancient Oak: I love the end of T. S. Eliot's poem *Four Quartets*. It is an epic poem that I have visited and revisited so many times. At the end he reminds us that every end is also a beginning and that every moment is where we start from.

The Barefoot Professor: And don't take our word for it. Enjoy exploring these ideas that every moment is an end, a death even, a beginning, a birth even. It's a miraculous idea.

Your mindfulness practice is where you practice what you need to live well. Your life is where you put mindfulness into practice. My hope is that the ideas in this book have become a lifelong friend at your side. I see the Barefoot Professor, Ancient Oak, Sam, Mohammed, Ling, and Sophia in you, me, and all of us. We are doing the best we can, falling into holes and climbing out again, finding beauty in the muddle, learning which streets to walk down and which to avoid, trying to be a good friend to ourselves, our friends, family, and the world we live in. People say, Willem, sometimes you don't seem that mindful. I laugh, but I'm serious when I reply, my life could have followed a very different trajectory. What I hope is that these ideas and practices are interesting and enjoyable, so they become something you make a part of your life, for life. That they help you live well. That they help all of us create not only the kind of world we'd like to live in but also the kind of world in which all those who follow us can flourish.

Resources

The 12 chapters of *Mindfulness for Life* have covered the foundational ideas and practices that I hope can resource you to live your life as you imagine. Throughout the chapters I signposted key resources to support you, and to make them as accessible as possible they are all available in one place.

The Mindfulness for Life Website: *mindfulnessforlife.uk*

This website has all the resources you need to deepen and extend your learning. What will you find there?

- An introduction to each of the 12 foundational mindfulness for life topics
- All the mindfulness practices
- Ways to support your learning, including mindfulness teachers, local groups, websites, books, films, and podcasts

In short, everything you need to integrate these ideas into your life.

A Trilogy of Books on Ancient Wisdom Meeting Modern Psychology to Address the Challenges in the Contemporary World

This book is part of a trilogy that together outline how contemplative traditions and modern psychological science can provide a way to live well in the contemporary world. The first, *Mindfulness: Ancient Wisdom Meets Modern Psychology*, I cowrote with Christina Feldman. Christina and I suggest that when ancient wisdom and modern psychology come together, they are no longer a set of ideas or practices but an illumination that guides us to live well in the contemporary world. We wrote it for mindfulness practitioners and teachers so that their learning and teaching could be informed by a deep understanding. That book was 10 years in gestation, 3 years in writing, and was published in 2019.

A forthcoming book, cowritten with Paul Bernard and Ruth Baer, is a specialist book for mindfulness teachers wishing to teach mindfulness courses. It's a how-to teachers' guide, with session-by-session guidelines, instructions for leading mindfulness practices, and much else. It draws on a rich lineage of mindfulness-based interventions developed by Jon Kabat-Zinn, Zindel Segal, Mark Williams, and John Teasdale, as well as many psychological scientists and contemporary mindfulness teachers.

All three books have in common the same basic purpose: offering mindfulness training as a guide to live well.

A Final Word

To make this book as accessible as possible, and against my instincts as a scientist, there are no references to clutter up the text. However, the two sister books reference all the source authors, books, and papers. The website also includes a downloadable document, *Mindfulness and MBCT Key Resources*. This includes references and links to many of the most important scientific papers and texts. Both the website and the key resources are updated regularly.

Index

About the Author

Willem Kuyken, PhD, is the Ritblat Professor of Mindfulness and Psychological Science at the University of Oxford, United Kingdom, and Director of the Oxford Mindfulness Centre. His work focuses on preventing depression, promoting mental health, and flourishing across the lifespan. Dr. Kuyken has published more than 150 journal articles and has been named one of the world's most highly cited researchers. He lives in London.